Living Longer, Living Better

Living Longer, Living Better

Adventures in Community Housing for Those in the Second Half of Life

Jane Porcino

CONTINUUM · NEW YORK

1991
The Continuum Publishing Company
370 Lexington Avenue, New York, NY 10017

Printed in the United States of America

Library of Congress Cataloging-in-Publication Data

Porcino, Jane.
    Living longer, living better : adventures in community housing
for those in the second half of life / Jane Porcino.
        p.   cm.
    Includes bibliographical references.
    ISBN 0–8264–0496–0.—ISBN 0–8264–0497–9 (pbk.)
    1. Aged—Housing—United States. 2. Communal living—United
States. 3. Shared housing—United States. I. Title.
HD7287.92.U5P67   1991
363.5′946′0973—dc20   90–41474
                                                              CIP

I dedicate this book to my husband, Chet, and my daughter Jeanne, whose loving and loyal support throughout the years of writing made it all possible.

This book is also dedicated to the rest of my family, which has grown to number seventeen. To Mary, Ann, John, Paul, and Vicky and their partners Amy, Malcolm, Christina, Marilyn, Michael, and Frank—and to my three special grandchildren: Matthew Joseph, Christina Jane, and Brooke Jane.

Acknowledgments

I am grateful to the hundreds of people in this country and abroad who have shared portions of their lives with me through long letters and hours of conversation in the warmth of their homes. Most of their names can be found alongside their exciting stories.

Special thanks go to my daughter Jeanne, who spent days of her busy life reviewing each chapter; to my husband, Chet, who was my travel companion as I crisscrossed the country interviewing; to my "Australian" daughter, Ann, who urged me to write this book and contributed interviews and encouragement.

And finally I want to thank Werner Mark Linz, the chairman of Crossroad/Continuum for recognizing the importance of this topic; my publisher, Michael Leach; my editor, Kyle Miller; and all the friends, relatives, and colleagues who offered their continuous love and support.

Contents

Preface

The ideas for a book on creative community living have been evolving since the completion of my book *Growing Older, Getting Better*. Its chapter on housing options and life-style transitions just touched on the topic, and yet this section provoked tremendous discussion and enthusiasm among readers and reviewers—and among the audiences I have lectured to around the United States.

For the past few years, I've been conducting workshops and surveys, lecturing and interviewing people in many states, and contacting national housing organizations. I eventually discovered that an informal, nationwide housing network does exist. There are many individuals and groups concerned about developing new housing options for the rapidly increasing number of those in the second half of life. A growing group of people have begun to investigate cooperate living arrangements, creating ways to meet both their personal housing and community needs. It is their stories that I share in this book.

It is resoundingly clear to me that many of us are focusing on where, how, and with whom we will spend our middle and later years. More and more people are seeking alternatives not provided by traditional housing arrangements, and yet there are few new design models of community living in this country. Concerned people have had to strike out on their own to develop the lifestyles they want in their "third age." As the aging population grows and doubles, new housing options will be necessary to meet the changing needs of these "feisty" generations in their forties, fifties, sixties, seventies, and eighties.

As a gerontologist, my search for housing/life-style options has both a professional and a personal basis. My husband and I are in our middle sixties—with many siblings, six adult children, and three grandchildren. Three years ago we sold our suburban home of twenty-seven years and moved into a New York City apartment; our youngest child, Victoria, is about to leave home.

At this point, we are in the midst of creating a supportive community with three or four other couples living in our complex. This group shares a common political ideology. We have fun when we go out together and have committed ourselves to being there for one another in any emergency. But still, we think and plan for the future—a future in which one of us may be living alone and perhaps unable to afford a city apartment. We are among the rapidly growing group of older people who want to build an extended family wherever we live, one that will offer us both independence and interdependence all the remaining years of our lives.

In the small town on Long Island in which I grew up, my family knew all of our neighbors, who supported and helped one another. Again, in the early years of our marriage, my husband and I felt connected with our neighborhood community. Everyone seemed to have a large family, and we all shared baby-sitting, personal problems, and emergency care. At that time, Chet and I were also part of a structured community within the Catholic Church called the Teams. This group of eight families had a common spiritual belief. They became our extended family. We formally committed ourselves to one another; to share joys and sorrows, to help in times of need, to share construction, gardening, and cooking skills, and to delight in each family's growth.

None of us had much more money than it took to raise a big family; and yet we were able to travel by caring for one another's children and staying in the homes of international Teams members around the world. I cannot imagine how we could have raised our family without the support of this community.

These experiences were also influential in the adult lives of our children. Mary left home after high school to do her "growing up" with a communal group of peers in Boston. Paul married and with his wife created an extended family, similar to the Teams, in Ohio. Jeanne and Ann surround themselves with supportive mother's groups as they raise our grandchildren. We all hunger for a genuine support network, knowing that it will help us live out our lives as fully and as vibrantly as possible.

The person who has most influenced my continuing thinking about cooperative living is my son John. His experiences have ranged from living with six siblings and sharing homes with college peers to his present intergenerational cooperative community in a bustling town in Massachusetts. John has always been determined to continue living in community. When he graduated from college, he traveled the country for many months, visiting several of the older international communities around the country. He wanted to see firsthand what they were like; their successes and their problems.

Several months ago, he and his new wife, Christina, began to plan a cooperative community in Massachusetts, based on a fifteen-year-old housing model which has been successful in many Scandinavian countries. This model, new to the United States, is called cohousing and is described in detail in chapter 4. It includes housing for couples and singles of all ages. Recently, John said to his father and me, "When you get tired of your new living arrangement in New York City, perhaps you would like to move into our community." Perhaps we will; it's a secure and satisfying thought for our old age.

Professionally, my interest in housing has continued to expand. In the early eighties, I was invited by New York's Governor Mario Cuomo to join his committee on aging and his task force on midlife and older women. The subcommittee on housing, which I chaired, recommended to the governor that women over fifty-five be surveyed about the type of housing they would like for their later years. Both committees began to realize that an appalling number of older women in New York State lived alone and were lonely.

To find out more, I cofounded the Group for Research on Midlife and Older Women. Our preliminary survey on transitions and stress in midlife and older women shows that the most stressful life event for them was change in their housing situations. Perhaps this is true because we are too timid, superstitious, or afraid to *plan ahead* in our lives.

I hope that this book will encourage people to develop their future housing plans before a major crisis or transition occurs in their lives. It is not a guide to specific communities (some excellent books containing this information are listed in the Bibliography and Resources section on page 181), but is written to shout to the world that there are *many* fulfilling options for housing and life-style changes as we age.

I anticipate people reading the book and saying, "This part of XYZ community is just what I am looking for, but I don't like the idea of this part of ABC housing." If readers can discover, through all of the examples presented, bits and pieces of what they need and want for their own futures, they can then begin to plan new ways of living in community and the means to enjoy fulfilled and zestful lives in their later years. For many, growing older can, and does mean getting better.

Introduction

Where we live and who we live with affect how we think, feel, and believe. A sense of home is central to our psychological well-being. We are all looking for a living environment that supports our autonomy, empowers us by accentuating our potential, and nurtures us. No area offers greater potential for creative change than that of housing and life-style.

This book is about some new ways people are choosing to live in their middle and later years. The people I have interviewed are either searching for or maintaining a life-style that offers them both privacy and community, more housing for less money, and social contact with those of similar interests, but of a mixture of ages. These people are creating new ways of thriving in their lives, rather than merely surviving.

A New Sense of Community Is Needed

This is especially exciting in consideration of the dramatic demographic changes that are taking place in our society, with some of the most radical changes occurring in longevity, family life, and work patterns. There are more midlife and older people in the world than ever before in the history of humankind. We are living thirty to thirty-five years longer than our parents or our grandparents at the beginning of this century, and women are living eight years longer than men. Widowhood or divorce leaves more than half of all American women alone in their later years, facing severe economic losses. The gap between the poorest and the richest in this nation has reached an all-time high.

Inflation, a rising number of one-parent families, the high rate of divorce, smaller and fragmented housing, and a growing isolation of both the young and the old has stimulated many people to search for alternatives to single-family suburban homes.

In the last fifteen years there has also been an unprecedented influx of women into the work force, many of them middle-aged and beyond. Women's earnings are two-thirds that of men's, leaving American women over sixty-five with a median annual income of only $6,500. Women of today are expected to work both in the labor force and in the home. Many of them are single women heads-of-households. Their large suburban homes require them to commute, and when they come home, they feel isolated from their communities.

So often, the changing needs of women (and of men in similar situations) have not been recognized by home builders. Little public attention and almost no governmental support are being given to devising a wide spectrum of housing options. Home designers need to begin developing smaller dwellings closer to work, with more shared facilities and improved public transportation.

Clearly, this country is in the midst of a major housing crisis, not only for women and the lower socioeconomic groups but for a majority of middle-class, middle-aged, and older Americans. An estimated one in three Americans—and 70 percent of Californians of all ages—are unable to afford their own homes. And yet, as we enter the twenty-first century, America is still without a national housing policy.

A nationwide public-opinion poll taken in 1988 indicates that millions of Americans were experiencing or concerned about housing problems, and that they wanted something done about them. Although some people prefer to live alone in their own homes, most fear loneliness (second only to poverty) as they age—

and are open to new ideas about life-styles. The Department of Housing and Urban Development (HUD) predicts that 50 percent of the American population will live in some form of shared facilities in the next twenty years.

New Definitions of Family

Already there has been a sharp increase in the number of households in which unrelated individuals live together. Transient work patterns have scattered family, relatives, and friends. And despite a government housing policy that continues to be based on the traditional nuclear family, friendship networks have had to begin replacing *family* networks in housing.

Even the definition of "family" has changed. A *New York Times* article that I recently read describes the need for a reformulated definition of family:

> How to define a family is becoming an increasingly important issue around the country. State governments struggle to determine how unrelated people living together—like the elderly, the handicapped, group homes for single people, and gay couples—fit into existing laws and regulations. Court cases continue to broaden the restrictions on the number of unrelated people living together as a "functional equivalent family." A court brief, filed in New York State's Court of Appeals recently, by religious leaders and other interested organizations, says: "While still perceived as an ideal for many, the nuclear family as the standard is now a myth."*

A New Understanding: Senior Housing for the 1990s

As we look into the future of housing for midlife and older Americans, we would do well to examine a new booklet published by the American Association of Retired Persons (AARP). It reports a

*April 27, 1989

LIVING ARRANGEMENTS OF PERSONS
65 + : 1988*

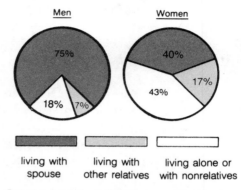

Men   Women

living with spouse   living with other relatives   living alone or with nonrelatives

Based on data from U.S. Bureau of the Census

Living Arrangements of Persons 65 +, 1988
From *A Profile of Older Americans*, AARP American Association of
Retired Persons.

survey of housing preferences, concerns, and needs, titled "Understanding Senior Housing for the 1990s." Fifteen hundred randomly selected adults (all over the age of fifty-five) were contacted by phone to determine how they perceived their current housing situation, and what they wanted for the future.

Three categories of aging people were identified: the "young old," age fifty-five to sixty-four; the "old," sixty-five to seventy-four; the "old old," over age seventy-five. Three categories of community housing were recognized: retirement housing or buildings planned for older adults; naturally occurring retirement communities (NORCs), in which most people have aged in place; shared housing, either with nonrelatives or with adult children.

The current housing arrangements of the respondents is as follows:

♦ 5 percent live in retirement communities.

♦ 27 percent live in NORCs.

♦ 43 percent have lived in their present home for over twenty years.

- 28 percent live alone (32 percent of women and 22 percent of men).

If the respondents were to move, they would:

- stay in the same city or county (63 percent).
- move within the same state (26 percent).
- move to a different state (11 percent).

They would most like to live:

- in a small town (34 percent).
- in the country (25 percent).
- in the suburbs (24 percent).
- in a city (13 percent).

When asked what type of housing they would most prefer—

- a surprising 86 percent said they wanted to stay in their present home and never move from there.
- 5 percent would prefer to move into an apartment environment that provides meals, housekeeping, transportation, and social activities.
- 3 percent would be interested in cooperative housing.
- 3 percent are considering moving in with a family member (22 percent of those surveyed said they were counting on their family to take care of them as they aged).

When asked with whom they would most prefer to live—

- 41 percent expressed a desire to live alone as they aged.
- 13 percent would entertain the possibility of moving into a cooperative house.
- 12 percent might share their home with nonrelatives.
- 17 percent would consider moving in with a family member.

A New Breed of Older People

People today are healthier, brighter, more longlived, and more energetic than ever before in history. Today's fifty-plus generation

Moving Destinations

Same city or county,
63%

Different city and county
in the same state,
26%

Different state,
11%

Base: 57
Source: Question 7b

Reasons for Moving

	Total %
Desire to change location	30
Home not suitable for my needs (too big, etc.)	18
Could not afford to stay in home	16
Health reasons (respondent)	7
Death of spouse	2
Wanted to move closer to family	—
Health reasons (spouse)	—
Other	27

Moving Destinations
Used with the permission of the American Association of Retired Persons
(AARP).

Tables on pages xx–xxiv are from *Understanding Senior Housing for the
1990s: An American Association of Retired Persons Survey of Consumer
Preferences, Concerns, and Needs,* 1990.

Urban/Rural Preferences

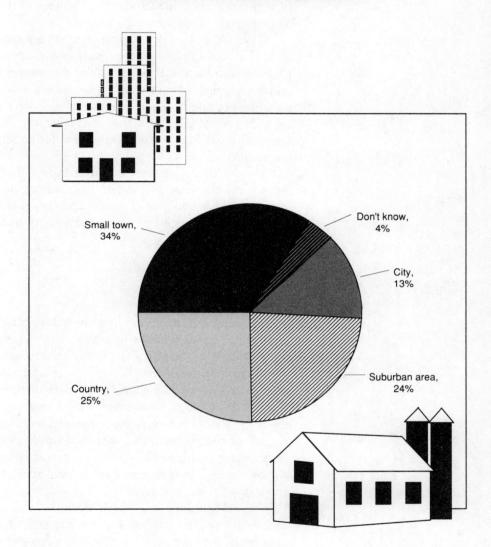

Urban/Rural Preferences
Used with the permission of the American Association of Retired Persons (AARP).

view midlife and aging with a sense of exhilaration and challenge and are determined to live full lives. This group are willing to break new ground, take risks, and make changes in their lives—indeed, to be pioneers for future Americans.

A small but growing number are ready to move away from the isolation of nuclear-family homes, private property, and rugged individualism. They want to take control of their later years and are saying; "I don't want to live in an old-age ghetto or even a middle-age ghetto—and above all else, I don't want to live alone or with one of my children." They are on the cutting edge of nontraditional living. They are reformulating ideas about living in community.

Housing literature written about this group commonly focuses on the frail and dependent elderly. It is time to begin focusing on the majority of Americans—vital and healthy individuals who are interested in new life-style options for the second half of life.

What Exactly Is Community?

In the beginning, everyone lived in tribes, small communities, or in large extended families in which they experienced unity with those who lived near them. Today, many areas of the country (particularly cities) have become large and impersonal, causing feelings of isolation and alienation in both our homes and our places of work. How often do you hear friends and relatives complaining about the lack of connectedness they feel in today's world? Seventy percent of the people questioned in a survey conducted by Daniel Yankelovich in his book *New Rules,* reported that they had many acquaintances but few close friends, and they experienced this as a serious void in their lives.

M. Scott Peck, in his recent book *A Different Drummer,* says, "All over the country there is the lack of, and the thirst for community. It may no longer be so pardonable to yearn for community without doing something about it. We humans hunger for genuine community . . . because it is the way to live most fully, most vibrantly."

How is community defined? *Webster's Dictionary* says the word comes from the Latin *communitas,* meaning "fellowship"—or

Neighborhood/Building Preferences

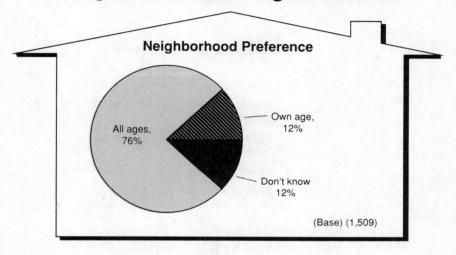

Neighborhood Preference

All ages, 76%

Own age, 12%

Don't know 12%

(Base) (1,509)

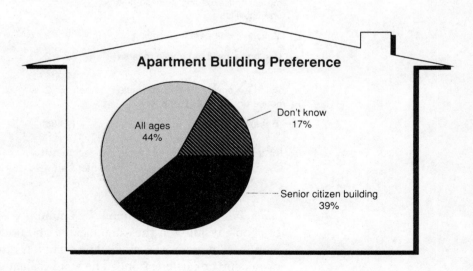

Apartment Building Preference

All ages 44%

Don't know 17%

Senior citizen building 39%

Neighborhood/Building Preferences
Used with the permission of the American Association of Retired Persons (AARP).

Interest in Alternative Living Arrangements

	Have Done %	Are Considering %	Would Consider %
Share home with one or more non-relative	15	2	12
Move in with family member	11	3	17
Obtain a second mortgage based on home equity	8	1	5
Move into a household shared by non-relatives	7	2	9
Modify home to include extra apartment	5	2	8
Move to home with unrelated person and pay rent in return for services such as meals, housekeeping, or personal care	3	2	10
Move into apartment that provides meals, housekeeping, transportation, and activities	2	5	32
Move into co-operative housing	2	3	13
Use home equity to obtain reverse mortgage	2	2	9
Purchase or rent small, removable house on relative's property	2	2	8
(Base)	(1,488)	(1,176)	(977)

Interest in Alternative Living Arrangements
Used with the permission of the American Association of Retired Persons (AARP).

communis, meaning "common." Community is defined as "a group of people residing in the same locality and under the same government . . . a group or class having common interests . . . common ownership or participation." The word *commune* is listed as "a small group of people, often in a rural area, whose members have common interests and share or own their property jointly."

In the last decade, the definitions of community have been modernized to meet our changing life-styles. Community is often viewed as the friendship and acquaintance networks replacing some of the historical functions of family in today's world. Some of the more recent descriptive writings about community sound like traditional definitions of the family, as does this one by Daniel Yankelovich: "Community evokes in the individual the feeling that 'Here is where I belong, these are my people, I care for them, they care for me, I am part of them, I know what they expect from me and I from them, they share my concerns. I know this place, I am on familiar ground, I am at home.'"

In a world of individual freedom, many of us yearn for a greater sense of connectedness—to really touch others and to experience a sense of unity with them. If we share similar activities and pursuits, we have the potential for building community with our family, friends, coworkers, neighbors, and even strangers. But community living both attracts and frightens people. It is not easy to give up the secure routine of an established life-style, to join with others. An even stronger reality, however, is that too many of us feel fragmented—disconnected from family and friends, with work lives at odds with our spiritual values. Of concern to many is the memory of the hippie communes of the sixties with their beliefs in free living, open sex, and drug use. Those life-styles simply didn't work and have all but disappeared. Today's new communities are totally different. In their short history, they have succeeded in creating loving, extended families just as real as the nuclear families that, for many people, no longer exist.

Why Do People Choose to Live in Community?

A ninety-year-old architect and suffragette I know, who lived for thirty years in community, says: "Living alone is not a human way to live. You come home to a dark house, cook your own dinner, eat by yourself. You go to bed by yourself, and you get up by yourself. It's just not a human way to live." A fifty-year-old I interviewed said: "I expect to live another thirty-five years. Alone? The idea terrifies me!"

These thoughts echo those of others I interviewed around the country and of people I talk to every day who are searching for community.

The early communes attracted mostly young people. Today, more mature and professional people are joining. Most are college educated and work in a wide variety of white- and blue-collar jobs. This is the first generation of midlife and older people considering community living—and being accepted by the community. Communities are just beginning to wake up to the benefits of having older people live with them. This seems to be due to two reasons: The initial founders are growing older themselves, and they are recognizing that people today are living longer lives, are healthier throughout their lives, and can be productive as long as they live.

This is the philosophy of Bob Brown, the founder of Clairmont Project, an intentional community in California: "It's obvious to anyone who has given any thought to the issue, that retired persons have a lot to offer community life and more time and love to contribute than most younger persons. It seems equally apparent that any community will be more stable and healthy the broader its spectrum of age."

The primary reason some people choose to live in community is to avoid living alone, which is difficult and unappealing to people of all generations. As they discover new ways to escape the loneliness of everyday life, people are also finding the emotional- and social-support networks they've found so difficult to establish in the outside world. One of the rallying cries of both the young and old in today's society is, "Where can I meet people?"

Community living gives people a greater measure of emotional security and stability in their lives. It makes continued independence possible, along with the interdependence with other committed and supportive people. Friendship, perceptions, feelings, compassion, and love are shared. The need for experiencing a greater intimacy with others is met in the new form of extended families. Others seek community to heal their spirit in times of personal crisis, such as widowhood, divorce, a last child leaving home, loss of a job, retirement, chronic mild illness, or the strain from caring for dependent aging parents.

Another major reason for living in community is to ease financial stress. People want and need to share the economic burdens of surviving in the world. When costs of land, housing, food, supplies, and resources are shared, people are able to find affordable and appropriate housing in areas they would otherwise not be able to live in. They can share the everyday process of living with others in a "richer" environment, with more attractive physical surroundings and intellectual stimulation. When people spend less money for basic living costs, they have more money for travel and leisure activities. Community living helps people of all ages to use the resources of the world more wisely and more efficiently.

As people learn the skills of relating and living with a diverse group of others, they begin to experience a deep bonding with new friends. They pool individual skills, such as cooking, fixing cars, repairing electric appliances, and sewing; they teach one another. The end result is an optimum physical and emotional environment. Sharing responsibilities gives people a feeling of self-worth. In many communities, older, retired people keep a watchful eye on children returning from school—and young parents contribute "pet- and plant-sitting" when older people are traveling. A measure of security is felt by all, since there is safety in numbers. By exposing themselves to a wider spectrum of thinking, individuals are encouraged and stimulated to continue growing in their own lives. A retired businessman says that living in community keeps him aware, flexible, and lively: "I have no time to become rigid or to congeal."

People also savor the luxury of the time-saving aspects of community—fewer responsibilities to cook, clean, and perform household chores. They enjoy having dinner prepared, having others to eat it with, and having someone to care when they are ill. Often, amenities such as computers, saunas, hot tubs, TVs, and sewing machines are shared.

The real delight is living with understanding, committed, and fun-loving people who share positive visions, common values, interests—and hope. Emotionally, it just doesn't make sense for people to continue living alone.

If we have the desire to try community living, we should be encouraged by M. Scott Peck's words: "In my experience only two individuals out of roughly five thousand could not be successfully incorporated into the community-building process." My own research shows that people all over the country have begun to take personal action to initiate independent housing alternatives. It is predicted that community living/shared housing will be the fastest growing housing design in the decades ahead.

Chapter One

The Process of Building Community: An Overview

Different Types of Communities

Alternative communities have been formed in every one of the industrialized countries around the world, including Israel, Australia, New Zealand, England, Scotland, Canada, Holland, Denmark, Sweden, Finland, Norway, Germany, India, Nigeria, Costa Rica, and the United States. Denmark has the largest number, with more than ten thousand established alternative communities.

The many ways people share life-styles and housing in these communities range from one-to-one shared housing and small-group living to large intentional communities. They include:

Accessory Apartments, a complete, new living unit installed in a single-family home—often for an older parent.

Cluster housing, any arrangement of homes clustered around a communal open space—small enough so that they don't look institutionalized, yet large enough for shared facilities to be possible.

Cohousing, a form of "living communities" based on the very successful villages found in many Scandinavian countries. A group of people purchase land together, build their own separate homes and a large community house. Residents of all ages come together in the desire for a more practical and social home environment. Based on democratic principles, the community has no professional management; instead, each resident serves on an interest-group committee.

Collaborative housing, private, self-contained housing units with extensive common areas and facilities. The housing is developed and managed by residents, with an emphasis on community.

Commune, unstructured group-living form popularized in the sixties, often built in rural areas.

Condominiums, an apartment building or housing area in which the living units are individually owned, with joint ownership of common areas.

Congregate housing, development-type housing, built and managed by private or public agencies, usually for the elderly in need of support services. Small private-living units share central dining areas, where meals are served.

Continuing-care communities, in which residents purchase a lifetime contract ensuring them housing, services, and medical care. In *life-care communities,* lifetime housing and total care is purchased for a substantial entrance fee plus monthly payments. Services may include meals, housekeeping, transportation, recreation, and health and nursing services. Sponsorship can be through a private developer or a nonprofit organization. *Enriched housing* provides subsidized congregate housing and support services for low-income, frail elderly.

Cooperative housing, a housing enterprise owned jointly by those who use its facilities or services. Residents purchase shares in a co-op corporation.

ECHO housing, temporary living units for older people, installed on the property of an adult child's home.

Home-sharing, a housing alternative offering living space to a nonrelative, in a single-family home—or groups of people renting or purchasing a home together. The people involved agree to share a dwelling space, home life, household expenses, responsibilities and, sometimes, social activities. *One-to-one sharing* involves two compatible, unrelated people living together in one of their homes or apartments.

Intentional communities, a group of people who choose to live cooperatively, because they share common values and a common purpose. Land, housing, and resources may be shared or owned individually.

Small-group living, two or more unrelated people sharing dwelling space and household expenses and responsibilities.

Retirement communities, apartments or homes for midlife and older people, most often located in suburban or rural areas. Individual homes are purchased, and common spaces such as a clubhouse or health club are shared. Outside space is maintained by the management.

Individual Considerations

As people think about community living, the most important consideration is who they want to live with. Some are looking for people their own age or of their own sex. Others are searching for an intergenerational group. Compatible people usually share a common belief system—religious, political, ideological, or cultural.

People need to decide what kind of space they will require, and where they want to live. Some function best in an urban environment, whereas others want the peace and quiet of a rural area. Other considerations may include proximity to family and friends, or climate.

Neighborhood services such as public transportation, nearby shopping, medical facilities, or a religious center may also be important priorities in making independent community living successful.

Those seeking community life-styles need to be stable— able to balance both private and social time in their lives. Above all, they should have a strong sense of their own self-worth. They need to be able to connect positively with others and to work out personal differences through a mutually agreed-upon process. They are often looking for new alternatives to marriage, the nuclear family, materialistic life values, and/or living alone.

The Process of Building a New Community

All that it takes to start a new community is one or two people who are really committed to doing it. They will need to persevere, with patience and dedication, in the hard work of the building process. The initial group may be small, but their first task is to be clear about their goals and purposes. Then they are ready to seek out others.

Finding compatible people is the most important part of the process and perhaps the most difficult. To find people who will be drawn to the idea of living in community, the founders usually start with friends who share common life values. The group can be expanded by word of mouth or by placing a newspaper ad inviting interested strangers to a meeting.

Innovative Housing of California, a nonprofit group in the Bay Area, initiates a regular series of workshops to organize groups of people interested in developing models of cooperative living. Slides are shown of successful cohousing communities in Europe. With the help of a facilitator, participants are asked to discuss their individual economic circumstances, needs, goals, and dreams about living in community. Equally important is asking each person what they will have to offer to a new community. The group has already leased or purchased more than seventy shared homes.

Active participation in the process of building community is necessary from the very beginning to create a closer and more supportive group. Inclusion of people of all ages and outlooks ensures that the community will be diverse; yet, a certain homogeneity in backgrounds, beliefs, life-styles, incomes, educational levels, and political philosophies is usually necessary. Participants need to be patient, willing to listen, and able to get things done. It is important to establish a process for reaching solutions through group consensus. When the relationships within the group are positive, the details will fall into place.

It may take several months of meetings to determine which people are really interested in moving ahead, and whose personalities are compatible. This group should be comprised of positive thinkers who will work with a sense of optimism and flexibility in the months ahead. In this process called *community building*, people are learning to trust one another and to create, through their emotional and social binding, the essential group spirit.

An equal distribution of responsibility and power should exist from the beginning. Working groups may be formed, and if the group is large, a core planning group might be chosen. The core group finds a large home or land site, works out the details of cooperative funding, and coordinates the hiring of an architect and building professionals.

The next major step is either buying the land together and/or finding the right piece of land to buy cooperatively and build on. There are several legal options for land ownership, ranging from having a single owner or small group purchase the land to a land trust, in which a corporation is set up to purchase land that is then rented to the community.

The design of this new community needs to bring people together on a daily basis. Common meeting spaces, play areas, and shared gardens should be part of the physical structure.

It is estimated that it will take two to five years from the first gathering of interested people before the final move into a new community.

Judging a Successful Community

As my husband and I visited communities around the country, it soon became apparent that the ones which seemed successful welcomed us with joy and an openness of spirit; there was a quickly felt sense of friendship. Though formal tours were arranged, we were encouraged to go anywhere we liked, see the types of living spaces, and talk to the residents. We were invited to share meals, attend services, and examine descriptive literature. There was a noticeable lack of tension in the daily work of the residents. We observed a uniqueness in each personal living space and a beauty and homeyness in the common shared areas and the outside environment.

One large intentional community invited all its women residents over forty years old, to spend an evening with me, openly sharing both their enthusiasms and problems. They talked about an ongoing personal and group process in their present life-style. Each woman felt she had been accepted as she really was, without needing to put on the different masks so many of us use in our daily lives. There was a strong interest in individual growth and fulfillment *and* the growth of the community.

Other characteristics that we found inherent in successful communities were:

+ a common identity that binds people together.

+ joyfulness—but also a sense of reality.

+ an evolving structure with clear rules decided upon and obeyed by the group.

+ residents' obvious thoughtfulness toward one another.

+ a safe environment in which people can speak and be heard; in which their ideas are valued, appreciated, and accepted; where individual differences are accepted.

- residents who frequently ask themselves how they are doing, and whether they are attaining their goals and keeping the original spirit of community.

- a group of people who can resolve conflicts without destructive physical or emotional trauma. This may involve decision making by consensus or any other method that works for a particular community. Often, trained mediators will assist in the process.

- residents who have been trained in cooperative living and who share responsibility for management, finances, and chores.

- an environment conducive to personal fulfillment and growth.

- excitement and a sense of adventure.

Chapter Two

Small-Group Living

Today, a growing number of pioneering midlife and older people are closing the doors on traditional living arrangements and are choosing to share their lives with small groups of nonrelatives. Small-group living is an old idea whose time has come.

The dynamic women and men I interviewed for this chapter were searching for three things: adequate housing, personal privacy, and independence/interdependence. Each was determined to make their own decisions about how and where they would live, to have control over their lives, and to explore new ideas and life-styles.

What Is Small-Group Living?

Small-group living involves two or more unrelated people sharing dwelling space and household expenses, and responsibilities.

New types of families are being created, combining privacy and companionship in a supportive, friendly environment where the sharing of housing and living costs can stretch dollars and promote the well-being and independence of the sharers. Small-group living offers a wide variety of options, of ownership or rental styles, and of managerial responsibilities. It works best when there is a mutual understanding of the sharing, along with some explicit rules that can be adjusted over time.

Small groups may be living in suburban split-level homes or cottages, urban town houses, high-rise apartment buildings, large, old farmhouses, or garden-apartment complexes. Most are within walking distance of shopping or reliable transportation.

What Is the History of Sharing Homes?

Small-group living is a new twist to an old concept. Past generations of Americans have a history of shared housing. At the turn of the century, an estimated 15 percent of the population lived with non-relatives. The early immigrants opened their homes to relatives and friends. There was always enough room to squeeze in "cousin Joe, just until he gets a job and can afford his own space"—a process that often took a year or more. People often opened up their homes to nonfamily individuals who were temporarily homeless. Some took in boarders to make ends meet. During the Depression, it was common to double up. Space magically expanded, as did love and support!

The number of people living with nonrelatives in America dropped considerably after World War II, because of the boom in construction and easy financing. The nuclear family became a firmly rooted tradition, with each family treasuring their own home, yard, and privacy. At the same time, corporations began to move employees and their families all over the country.

Today, with higher rents, smaller families, and the lack of federal support for low-income families, shared housing has made a sharp comeback. In 1987, an estimated fifteen thousand people were placed in small shared housing by some four hundred home-matching agencies throughout the country (up from only forty organizations working in the field in 1981). Small-group living is an incredibly cost-effective way of creating housing—with average monthly rents from three to five hundred dollars. Private and non-profit matching agencies estimate that they can place an individual in shared housing for about five hundred dollars.

Small-group living has proven so successful that it has made its way into the media. "Golden Girls," the popular TV show, is a good example. It depicts the successes and problems of four older women sharing a home. I recently interviewed Rue Mc-Lanahan, who stated that her part in the show was based on personal life experience. Several years ago she shared her home with another woman and a child. This program and others like it are sending out the positive message that shared life-styles can be fun—and beneficial for all concerned.

What Kinds of People Can Be Expected to Share?

> Many older people don't want, or can't afford, to live in special retirement communities, and they also don't want to live alone. It can be lonely rattling around in a big house all by yourself: there is no one to debate the news with, no one to cook breakfast for, no one to steady the stepladder while you change the light bulb. And for many of the 30 percent of today's elderly who live alone, a big apartment or house can be very hard to keep up. Living alone denies millions of older men and women the friendship, support, and love that can come from sharing a home with a loved one or with family members. Since not all older people have the luxury of available relatives to live with, several clever solutions, such as roommate matching and shared housing, have begun to pop up all over the country.
>
> Ken Dychtwald, *Age Wave*

Small-group living is appropriate for anyone who enjoys being with people, communicates well with others, is flexible and open-minded, finds living alone unappealing, and who needs housing and companionship. People who are *not* right for shared living are those who are fussy, rigid, and demanding in their daily-life patterns or those who have emotional problems.

Small-group living can be effective for people of all income levels. Individuals can choose to live with peers (with midlife or older people exclusively) or as an intergenerational "family," open to all without regard to age, sex, marital status, or physical disability.

I interviewed many people who were successfully living in a form of small-group housing. About half of them had a lifelong commitment to the group they were living with. They reported that sharing a home with this group had brought them economic security, companionship, an exchange of services, and freedom from isolation. The others also believed strongly in the ideals of small-group living but saw their present home as only one stage in a lifetime series of shared living experiences, or *serial shared living.*

In 1987, 35 percent of people placed in small, shared homes by matching agencies were over age sixty-two. Maggie Kuhn, the eighty-four-year-old founder of the Gray Panthers, has lived in small-group housing for twenty-five years. She says, "It brings together people who live alone and are fearful. It makes loneliness obsolescent."

What Are the Variations in Living Arrangements?

There are as many variations in space-sharing designs as there are people creating them. You can invite one or more people to share your home, form a group of people interested in buying and sharing a large home, or you can move into an already existing small-group home.

Economics plays a major factor in design. Those who can afford it may arrange for a spacious, private bedroom (large enough for conversation/eating/study and sleeping), as well as their own private bathroom and kitchenette. For others who are concerned about finances, a private bedroom space and shared common area suffices.

In small-group housing arrangements, the following kinds of spaces might be shared: living-room and dining-room space, lounge/TV room, a working kitchen, bathrooms, guest rooms, recreation and storage areas, garage or parking space, or a garden.

What Are the Benefits of Small-Group Living to the Sharers?

Physical, economic, health, safety, psychological, and social benefits make sharing not only more affordable but desirable. For many it is easier to get along with a family-size group than with forty or more people sharing lives in some of the larger intentional communities.

Group members who care will act as an extended family. Household chores and rent or carrying charges are shared, relieving financial stress and allowing participants to enjoy a few "extras"; health improvement results as sharers assist one another through minor crises and illnesses; isolation and loneliness are alleviated; people feel safer and more independent.

How Does Small-Group Living Benefit the Community?

When small groups of unrelated individuals join forces and share a common space, it benefits them and the community at large. More housing is available for younger families, homes are kept in better repair, there is a reduced need for support services, and the cost to the community of nursing-home care is cut in half.

Small-group living is for people of all ages who wish to live with others instead of living alone. It can be an exciting adventure, with the potential for enriching the lives of all concerned.

Types of Small-Group Living Arrangements

Most small-group living arrangements fit into five categories. The first is one-to-one shared housing.

One-to-One
Shared Housing

Today, three quarters of the population over age sixty-five own their own homes, and many choose to stay in their homes despite loneliness and financial difficulty. However, their houses are often too big, too costly, or inappropriate for their present-day needs. There are thousands of unused rooms in older people's homes. Many Americans—young and old alike—are looking for low-cost housing. One way they are getting together is through one-to-one shared housing—two compatible people living together in one of their homes or apartments.

Sometimes, people arrange this type of living privately by word of mouth or a discreet ad in the local newspaper. A growing number of governmental, private, and nonprofit matching agencies around the country have made the process easier and safer. A lonely homeowner who is financially stressed may be matched with a person who is searching for affordable shelter. Professional social workers, screening for financial and personality considerations, help make good and lasting matches. Detailed screening questionnaires include views on pets, children, smoking, alcohol, religious preference, and hobbies. Follow-up arrangements include telephone calls and visits between the participants. There is no rule against pairing members of opposite sexes: however, the majority of applicants are women seeking other women. Matching agencies will also help negotiate a shared-living contract between participants, provide follow-up counseling, and make appropriate referrals to related government agencies about entitlement programs.

There is no one right way to share a home. Some people are looking for an extended family situation in which they can share meals and social activities. Others choose one-to-one sharing so that they will have more time to work in a busy job, to travel, or to gain more financial freedom. Still others are looking for a strictly tenant/landlord relationship in which private space is rented for a fee, and some common areas are shared.

Zoning laws remain a problem in areas of the country where it is illegal for unrelated people to live together. However, variances have increasingly been awarded to people over sixty who wish to open their homes to sharers or renters. This is especially true when the sharer provides some services that will allow the homeowner to remain in his or her familiar surroundings for many more years.

In a few cases, despite careful screening, the one-to-one matching arrangements fail, usually because of personality conflicts. However, most matches have been successful in satisfying the companionship and financial needs of the participants. Firm friendships have developed between the new companions, as well as with family members, on both sides. In the end, it is the chemistry as well as the contract that make home-sharing work.

One-to-one success stories abound. A widow wanted to keep her rambling house that, though uneconomical to maintain, was full of memories. It had become too quiet, with empty rooms and silent meals. She was matched with a retired teacher eager to move from her apartment, where rents were skyrocketing. They both say, "We couldn't be happier and more compatible if we were sisters."

A retired couple who were desperately afraid they would lose their home because of rising taxes and fuel and utility bills, found a congenial person to rent one room to bring in the extra money they needed. And a divorcée I interviewed says, "I not only found a room but a real friend and companion. We go shopping together and share vacation trips."

Student Sharers

Frequently, students are matched with appropriate families and exchange household services for a reduction in room-and-board fees. They often do light or heavy housework, cook, take care of yard maintenance, or act as a companion for an older person. These are short-term living situations, lasting from one academic year to the entire time that the student is studying.

California University of Pennsylvania offers one of a growing number of nationwide programs that match students with others in the community. They have found that uniting college students with older people requires a careful matching of needs. All participants fill out a five-page application with questions ranging from their views on pets to pet peeves. The students visit their prospective roommates several times before a match is made.

One successful match was described in a recent *New York Times* article. A twenty-three-year-old college junior was matched with a ninety-seven-year-old woman—an unlikely couple to be sharing a home. The student enjoys the pleasures of living in a house instead of a dormitory. In exchange for a rent reduction, she does the shopping, mows the lawn, and performs other household chores. The homeowner is delighted to have a young person available in case of an emergency. "I wouldn't want to live any other way," says the young sharer. "We're friends and she's fun. I keep her up on modern times and she gives me history lessons."

A fifty-six-year-old widow I interviewed says: "I can foresee that I must change my life-style dramatically in order to survive financially. I love my house, garden, and spacious acreage and want to remain close to where I work. My decision is to rent rooms to college students.

"Two decades ago when my mother was widowed," she continues, "she declined to live with any of us. Instead she chose to stay in her large city apartment and rented her spare bedroom to two college students. When I asked her why she didn't get a roommate her own age, she said that older people were too rigid and settled in their ways. My mother would on occasion sew a button, hem a dress, cook—and the young women would help out with the grocery shopping. It was a wonderful experience for her. They truly shared, had freedom, and yet led parallel lives."

Family Home Conversions

The second type of small-group living arrangement is family home conversions. Many of the people I interviewed had converted their single-family home to share with several others. They all had to confront the rigid zoning laws developed in most American communities so many years ago—although, as housing options grow scarcer, local officials are increasingly aware of the need for shared housing for people of all ages and family status.

For six years I was able to observe closely the home in which my son John chose to live in community. We visited him

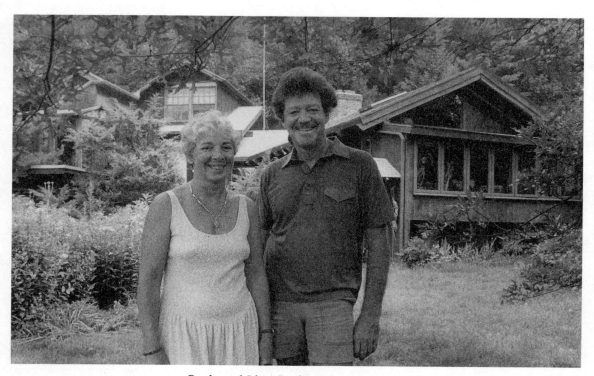

Prudy and Llan Starkweather in front of their home in Leverett, Massachusetts. Photographer: Martha Tabor, Working Images Photographs, Washington, D.C.

frequently, often spending the weekend. One Christmas vacation, ten members of our family gathered there for a joyful two-day reunion. Shortly after this, I interviewed Prudy, one of the owners.

PRUDY AND LLAN STARKWEATHER

Llan and I married twenty years ago. We had seven children ranging in age from a new baby to a twelve-year-old. We moved into a house in Leverett, Massachusetts, the central part of which Llan designed and built. The house is on ten acres of wooded land, has a lovely pond that we use for swimming and ice-skating, and a sauna.

There were two things I had dreams and fantasies about: adding extra rooms to the house and having extra adults around. However, whenever we built new rooms, they had to go to our family. Eventually, the kids began to move out. As each child left, they lost their room immediately. We rented it out. The "nest" was not emptied, it was immediately filled. We decided we liked it.

Right now, I think that the community here is the central focus of my life. The average age of our housemates is about thirty. We try to avoid people under twenty-five, and we have no upper age limit. Both Llan and I are in our fifties. We feel an agelessness here. It's a lot like family—but more of a utopian kind of family. We've done away with the old family patterns. Yes, people still do family types of things. You can find clothes in the middle of the living room, or dirty dishes in the sink. But now everyone is open to being reminded about things, and you don't get the kind of response you get as a mother. I try not to play the mother role.

It's somewhat harder being the homeowners. We have the overall responsibility for the house. Llan is very willing to do that, from repairing burners, to planting a garden, to making stained-glass windows. Without that, we would have to hire people to do lots of the work around the house. I handle all the finances. Rents range from one hundred and ninety to two hundred and forty-five dollars a month, depending on the size of the room and on the current rental rate in this area. Rent includes utilities, phone, washer and dryer—everything except food. At present we have two food-buying plans and two refrigerators. Whoever is home at night cooks their own meals and we eat together. Once in a while, one of us will cook a meal for everyone—and people often make loaves of bread or cookies for the house to share.

Who Does the Housework?

We have three work plans. One is for the kitchen (that's shared weekly with everyone except me; I'm the substitute), and we each take turns cleaning the common space every weekend. We also have two work days each year during which everyone is required to pitch in to do yard work, build a dock together, repair porch floors, clean all the windows in the house—jobs like that. We hold house meetings every couple of months to make major decisions or to resolve any problems people are having. Everyone owns and maintains their own car. We are eight people and one cat, and the group process takes over rather than the couple process.

Having a lot of people around is both good and bad. When you walk into the house, there are usually one or two other people there, which means that there is always someone to share with if you want to share. People are friendly and warm, and they care. That's the hard part too; it's sometimes difficult to be alone in the house. We've made an agreement that we can just say hi and walk through the room. When our doors are shut, we are not to be disturbed.

Living here means being involved with others' lives. I know lots about everyone who lives here, how their relationships and lives are going—and they know the same about me. Sometimes we all go out just for fun; last night we went for a jazz-boat ride down the Connecticut River, and we recently spent a weekend together in New York City. These things make for a better spirit in the house.

When someone is ready to leave (people tend to stay three or four years), everyone living in the house begins the interviewing process for a new person. We look for a spiritual quality. It can be pretty vague—it doesn't necessarily mean people going to church—but a quality you can feel. We look for someone with a relationship to the world and a "happy energy" (when certain people are around, all of our energy levels rise), but we also need quieter people for balance. If we're hesitant about someone, we ask them to come in for a trial period.

Llan and I have been doing this for eleven years and have had more than thirty different people living in our home. Our lives have a feeling of continuity, because we have our families living within fifteen miles of here. We continue to be involved with our parents, our children, and now, our first grandchild. We also feel a sense of continuity within the house. The comings and goings don't feel as disruptive as they did in the early years. When someone leaves, you have to go through a period of loss for a little while, and then you're busy paying attention to the person who is coming. Each time someone new moves in, there is a new dynamic, and you enjoy looking for that.

Advice for Others

You asked me what advice I would give to others about the kind of life-style we lead. They should first examine what they need and want in their lives. Women or couples who want to stay in their own homes could try it on a trial basis—slowly and somewhat carefully, to see if they like it. Each person needs to learn what works for them and what doesn't. You have to be willing to give up some things—some control. When your own kids are around, you still exert some control. So part of my advice would be to try it soon after your kids leave, before you get "cast in concrete."

Remember that you can change anything that's not right for you. Things should change when they're not working. Over the course of the years, we've changed our food-buying plan, and we choose housemates who have more of a feeling of being connected with the house.

People can be creative with this life-style. We have thought about selling shares in the house for people to continue living here. That's another way to do it.

This kind of living is good both economically and socially. The rents pay for the mortgage and all the ongoing expenses of the house. It has freed Llan and me from boring nine-to-five jobs. We have to earn only enough money for our food, and whatever else we want to do in our lives, such as travel. This is very liberating. Our way of life has allowed both of us to grow in new ways.

I wish my eighty-year-old mother would rent out a couple of her rooms, but she's just too rigid. When I look at my mother, I realize that I'm not really afraid of aging, but I am afraid of what this culture will do to me. Getting old or being decrepit or being in pain or discomfort for a year or two—that's a little scary to me. But mainly what I'm afraid of is people taking over my power—taking all my decision making away from me and sticking me someplace where I'd rather be dead. Control is a big issue for me right now.

This kind of living provides lots of change in our lives. If Llan and I were alone, we might tend to settle down—to grow and change less than we do now. I like what happens to us with lots of people around. I feel happy with my life, still knowing that someday in the future I might want to move on to another life stage.

I discovered another family-home conversion in Connecticut. Maintaining two small-group homes has been an economically sound and a socially exciting adventure for Fern Robinson, now in

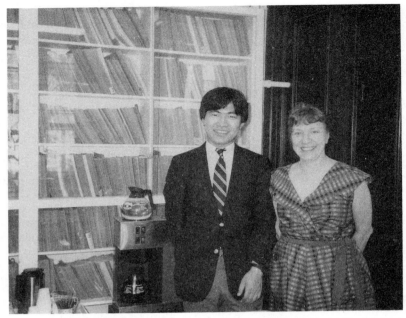

Fern Robinson, New Haven, Connecticut, with roommate Toshi from Japan.

her sixties. Sitting in the large, bright, and tastefully decorated living room in her home in New Haven, I was impressed by Fern's vitality, entrepreneurship, and warm hospitality.

FERN ROBINSON

This large house in New Haven, Connecticut, was my only "gift" when my marriage of thirty-one years ended in divorce. The financial aspects of the divorce were very difficult. I had no alimony, no permanent job, no retirement fund, and no real career. Most of my married life, I'd followed my husband around the world as he developed his expertise.

Thanks to the women's movement, I decided to return to school in 1973 to finish my bachelor's degree and earn a masters in political science. I have a secondary degree in education and sociology—so I am a certified teacher as well. I now teach English as a second language to welfare mothers, immigrants who need the English for jobs, and sometimes I teach in the prisons.

At the time of the divorce, my three adult daughters had already left home. I realized that I might be able to stay in my home and support myself if I rented out the entire house. So I started with six people, all from the Yale housing-office list. Since then, I've had housemates from all over the world and from every ethnic group.

With the new income coming in, I was able to pay the rent and all of my bills. Three years ago I bought the house next door. Now I have twenty-four rooms, all furnished from tag sales, people who were moving, and the things I've collected throughout the years. Everything is secondhand. Optimally, fifteen people live in these two houses. We share a kitchen, living room, bathrooms on each floor, dining room, large summer porch, and the yard. I have reserved three really private rooms and a bathroom for myself. Everyone else has a large bedroom. I keep the common rooms clean but get lots of help with the yard, garbage, and bathrooms. Everyone cleans up after meals. This house is well built, allowing for lots of quiet and privacy. We eat dinners together often. When I have guests for dinner, I usually invite anyone who is home. If they have someone in, they often do the same. We always say you should never feel obligated—only if you want to do it. It has worked out very well.

In the summer I charge three hundred and fifty dollars a month. Recently, I registered one house as a bed and breakfast, charging thirty-five dollars a night.

I haven't done anything about the zoning—I started off slowly and I just let it go. And not one neighbor has ever said anything to me about it. My houses are very quiet. My neighbors, in their large single-family homes, are all working. Here someone is always at home, which makes the neighborhood more secure. Maybe not asking is the best way to do it. My neighbors were amazed when I bought the second house. One of them, who is lonely living in her ten-room house, said to me, "I wonder who bought that house?" When I said I had, she said, "But I thought you were a poor divorcée." I said, "I am, but I just did it, and it's all right." She would be so much happier living like this. She lives in a world of fright, but always says, "I would never want other people living with me!"

People Keep Returning

People who have lived with me in the past are always showing up at the door. One is coming this week. She lived here when she was going through a life crisis. She was young and needed a mother figure. Many times I play the role of a mother. I often have to say, "Look, I'm really not your mother, but I can sometimes be your friend." But there were times when someone needed to be cuddled, when they were really on the brink. But I am also very good at referrals (I know so many people in town), so that their problem is placed in more professional hands. I don't have that much time.

People stay here from three weeks to three years, but for the *most part, it's a stopgap in people's lives. Most stay while they are in training at Yale, and then they move on.*

The average age here ranges from twenty to thirty-five. Phillipa, my Australian friend, is my age, as is a doctor from Iran who comes every year for three months. He feels like part of the fixtures now.

I took a risk when I bought the house next door, but I saw it as my one chance for a retirement and pension fund. My income is only fifteen thousand dollars a year, and so I asked my children to sign the deed with me. The price was two hundred and twenty-five thousand dollars, but now, three years later, it's worth three hundred and seventy-five thousand dollars. One thing I've learned in the last ten years is to gamble.

This is not a boarding house—it's much more. The scene changes all the time. We may have a group in the house that becomes very close. They'll have good times together, eat together, have parties together, and share in so many ways. That group may go, and the new group might be much more distant with one another.

The Gathering Time

We call this house "the Club," because people come from both houses to talk or watch TV together in the evenings. That's the gathering time when people share things. Last year we had a fun group. We had a run on doctors—a Korean, a German, a Mormon, and a young woman doctor from the United States, plus a medical psychologist, an architect, and a violinist with the Yale Symphony.

Everyone buys their own food, but they are a very sharing group. Two of my tenants are gourmet cooks. No matter what time they get home, they make wonderful dinners. They make so much food, that they always share with anyone around. That's the kind of thing we do in our house—extra things. The Mormon, Greg, was used to a big family, and he loved all the attention he got here. He'd stretch out on the couch—in the middle of all those people—and feel at home.

I'm always planning ahead for my next venture. My plans are to sell these two houses and buy a small house with one other person in my hometown of Pittsburgh. I'm starting life anew. For years I've been interviewing women all over the world about their roles in life—and I plan to write a book about it. I need a peaceful place to do that.

I have also considered moving to a Quaker retirement village in Maryland, which would enable me to travel and yet come back to community. I met some wonderful people living there when I went to Russia, and they want me to come visit. But I'm really a city person; it may be too rural for me.

I never feel lonely, and economically, sharing my homes has worked out well. It's been a busy and happy eight years.

Maggie Kuhn, eighty-five, who wrote the foreword to my book *Growing Older, Getting Better*, is a friend and colleague. She is the founder and national convener of the activist Gray Panther Movement in the United States. In her personal life as well as in her professional life, Maggie is one of this country's first advocates for intergenerational community living. Several years ago she converted her brownstone into a home for people of many ages.

MAGGIE KUHN

There are thousands of wonderful old people living alone in thousands of houses all over America. More often than not, they are lonely, isolated, and frightened. There are also thousands of younger people who would like to live with them, not as boarders, but as friends. I emphasize the word friends, *because that is what multigenerational living is at its best.*

Presently, I share my house in Philadelphia with seven people of different ages. We each have our own rooms and privacy, which we all respect. We also have common space to share, so we can be alone or together, according to our wishes. As it happens, we are all busy working, studying, organizing—and so we manage to have dinner together as a family only once or twice a month. My housemates pay rent and thus enable me to afford to live a bit better, and we all share housekeeping chores. We always have people around to teach us things, to pay attention to us, and to share with us. It is such a secure and fulfilling arrangement that I know it would be an ideal situation for others.

Buying/Renting a New Home for Small-Group Living

It is sometimes easier to find a "neutral" home or apartment for a group to live in—one which has no history for any of the participating members. This is the third type of small-group living.

Five to eight people seems to be an ideal household size, according to those who have experienced small-group living. Some groups decide to rent a home for a year or so to test their compatibility. Others decide to purchase the property as a group and jointly

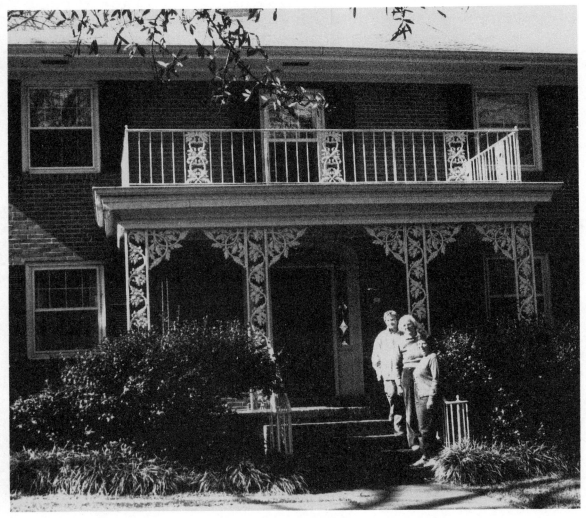

Members of The Molly Hare Cooperative, Durham, North Carolina.

build on it. Often, an underused large space like a school building, monastery, or loft may be converted.

It is more difficult to find sufficient space in an urban area in which to build small communities, but some people around the country have succeeded in doing so. Elizabeth Freeman, long interested in cooperative living, purchased a small apartment house near Duke University, in Durham, North Carolina. Neighbors and

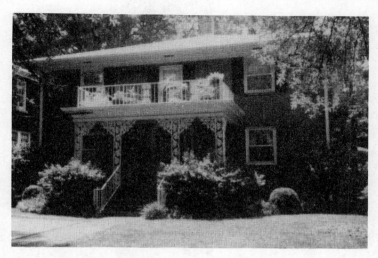

The Molly Hare Cooperative

A New Concept for Durham:

Cooperative Apartments designed to provide safe, companionable, affordable living.

Brochure for The Molly Hare Cooperative.

friends live together and have formed a new community within walking distance of shops and services. Presently, four women ranging in age from forty to eighty-three are living in what has been named The Molly Hare Cooperative. They each own their own modern, energy-efficient apartments, and two other units are being renovated. Membership in the cooperative costs between seven and nine thousand dollars (refunded should you decide to leave). Members hold lifelong occupancy rights, gain a tax deduction, and make a good investment. Monthly rents range from three hundred and sixty-five to five hundred dollars, depending upon the size of the apartment.

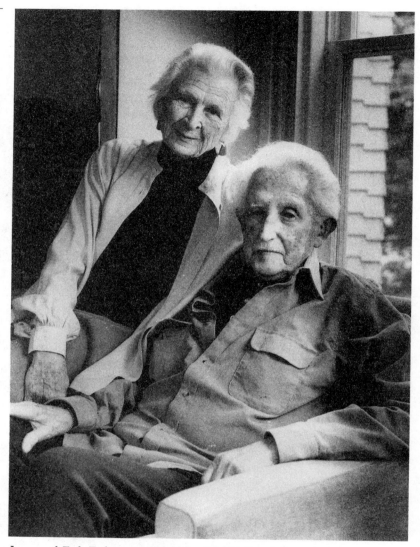

Joan and Erik Erikson, at home in Cambridge, Massachusetts.
Photographer: Sarah Putnam, *The New York Times.*

ELIZABETH FREEMAN

*This concept of cooperative housing seems an answer to many of
our problems. We have a hospitalized eighty-three-year-old housemate, and two of us are willing and able to help her get back to
health. The American tragedy is that so many older women are*

shipped off to nursing homes, when there is a possibility of coming home with caring others to help.

Some of the positive experiences of living in a small cooperative environment are: Sharing meals. Going out at night. Going to the movies, concerts, special events. Walking at dawn. Sitting on the porch and talking with members and neighbors. Cat- and dog-sitting. Mail retrieval while away. Working together on the yard—planting things and raking leaves. Preparing a stew for an ill friend. Planning and putting a banner across the driveway when a member returns from abroad. Sharing knowledge: gardening, cooking, decorating, art, carpentry, plumbing, electricity, sewing, and more. Hiking in the woods. Taking classes together. Reading and sharing food bargains. Putting up guests. A cleansing ceremony for one apartment. Birthdays and reunions. Helping out in times of illness or distress, accidents and operations. Loan of a car for repairs. Airport trips and doctors' appointments.

Joan and Erik Erikson (aged eighty-six and eighty-seven respectively) have recently purchased a gracious, large home in Cambridge, Massachusetts, with two professional women in their forties. All four have worked together for many years at the nearby Erikson Center. They allot an apartment to a young friend, a doctoral student, who does errands and some of the heavier tasks in the house. All five people are connected by work and similar interests.

The Eriksons, like many other married couples, enjoyed living on their own for many years after their three children left home. They had been spending eight months a year in a suburban California home and another four months in a rented apartment in Cambridge. Here they both wrote, taught at Harvard, and conducted research at the Erikson Center.

JOAN AND ERIK ERIKSON

Erik and I began to realize that we had lots of friends in California, most of whom worked during the day, whereas we were retired and writing at home. We were not close to libraries and stores and couldn't go anywhere without a car. We were ready for a change.

We thought for a while of going into a new retirement community in Santa Rosa. We looked at it very seriously and then realized that we would constantly be with people at least as old as we are. It wasn't for us. We like to have young people around; their spirit is important.

The more our two colleagues urged us to move to Cambridge and share a house with them, the more we thought it would be a good idea. Together, we began to look for a big old house close enough to walk to Harvard and the Erikson Center; we wanted to be independent of a car. We actually put a string down on a map to make a circle of the district we wanted.

We finally found this house, which was in terrible shape—but it is across from a park and a library and within walking distance of the university and the center. The four of us bought the house and paid for its rehabilitation. We spent a lot of time having it ripped up and redesigned to give us what we wanted—spacious and beautiful apartments for three single people and for ourselves.

We had a lawyer work out the details. Our own living spaces and furnishings belong to us, and we share a kitchen, living room and dining room. Each person has a good-size apartment with a small kitchen, bath, bedroom, and study. It's much less expensive with the four of us owning the house together and sharing the cost of utilities. Everyone takes care of their own space, and we hire a person to come in once a week to clean the common spaces. That way it doesn't get to be a hassle.

We're really like a family. We celebrate all "celebratable" things together. Our housemates have family and lots of younger and older friends, and so do we. Almost always when we use the common rooms, everyone is invited. Here, Erik and I feel a part of life—we don't feel shunted off somewhere. Our new "family" brings us their joys and sorrows, so we're not just muddling in our own. You could spend all of your time reminiscing in your old age, and that would be awful. I don't want to stop with the past—I want new things in my life. I attend courses, lectures, and workshops at Harvard all year long.

Goodwill is Required

There's so much that entails goodwill when you live in community. You can get huffy and persnickety lots of times, but you don't have to. I don't want to make it sound dreamy, because it's not, and you'd be misleading the world if you wrote that. Everyone has different ideas about practicality and efficiency. Sometimes for me that manifests itself in the kitchen, where I like everything in its place. Isn't it stupid how we all blow up about little things that don't amount to a hill of beans? You have to take distance from them and see where you're being unreasonable. Erik's frustration is with his hearing, especially when there are a lot of us around the dinner table.

I have energy and good health, although I'm slowing up a bit. Erik's health isn't as good as mine. He's hard of hearing, with *not as much energy, but he's not ill in any way. This is not a temporary living situation for any of us. We're here to take care of one another. We all belong to the Harvard Health Services, which means that we always have somewhere to go, twenty-four hours a day, if we're ill.*

I wrote something in my latest book about the attributes of wisdom and aging. We've got to inculcate them in people throughout life, so that everyone will be ready for old age when they get there. They include things like learning about interdependence, instead of this constant yacking we all do about independence. We are interdependent, and we're kidding ourselves if we think we are not. For an older person to think they can afford to grow older independently is nonsense. I think you also need to know your own capacities and use them appropriately for as long as possible—so that you don't take on that "I'm now old" mode and stop trying. But it does mean you have to have a realistic sense of what you can do. You have to be resilient, hopeful, and have a sense of humor. These are mandatory things for living together in any community, and the family is the place to start learning them. I love knowing what I want my adult kids to depend on me for, and what I don't; and what I can depend on them for, and what I won't.

I feel the plusses of the last two-and-a-half years are so much greater than any of the minuses. It's a good way to live for us— and possibly for many others.

Moving Into an Established Small-Group Home

Some people will be lucky enough to find a well-established small-group home. This fourth type of group living has been existing successfully for a decade or more. Whenever it has space, the group looks for a new housemate by "sending out the word" to friends and acquaintances or by putting an advertisement in an appropriate newspaper, journal, or on a local bulletin board (in universities, food markets, and bookstores). One person I know who was searching for a small-group home had a flat tire on his bike, went into a local laundry to use their phone, and there found an ad for the house he has lived in happily for the last six years. He calls it serendipity!

Applicants are usually screened by phone and personal interviews. After this process, a decision is made by those already living in the house.

The major advantage of moving into a well-established home is that most of the work already has been completed! You don't have to spend years building a new community. The residents have worked out their daily-life patterns, furnished the common rooms, and decided upon equitable rents, division of work, and a conflict-solving process. New members just have to fit into the already established norms. However, to some this may be a disadvantage. The rules and regulations have been set by others, and it might take time for your input to be considered.

Consider this successful example of a forty-five-year-old divorced woman living in a small-group home.

> *I've been living in a twelve-member family for the last five years. We live in an old twenty-five-room house in Berkeley, California. Each of us is single, aged eighteen to fifty-three. Four of us are middle-aged women. We cooperate in buying food, preparing meals, completing housekeeping chores, and maintenance. It's ecologically (as well as economically) sound to have two refrigerators, stoves, and washing machines rather than twelve. We even share our cars. I feel respected and valued by my housemates, nurtured in our sharing, caring family.*

Sue Koritz, a sixty-eight-year-old political activist, lives in a small-group home in Chestnut Hill, Massachusetts with eight other people, including a single mother with a three-year-old child.

> SUE KORITZ
>
> *I'd still be working and never would have been able to retire, if I didn't have this type of life-style. I have a small pension and a social-security check, with total assets of less than twenty-five thousand dollars, to last me the rest of my life. I love living here, and experiencing the sharing between generations. It keeps me open to things that are going on with younger people. They respect me because of my experiences. Right now I feel in control of my life and very serene.*

People of all ages and similar backgrounds have moved into established intergenerational small-group homes. One of them is sixty-two-year-old Betty Dexter, who lives in the oldest coop-

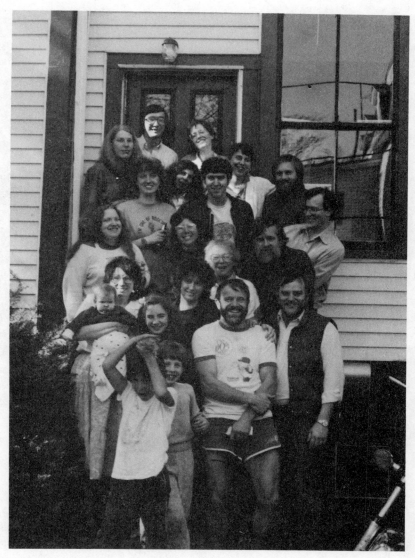

Sue Koritz and "family" in Chestnut Hill, Massachusetts.

erative house in Cambridge, Massachusetts. She has been divorced for twenty years and is the mother of five adult children. Betty has a bachelor's degree in art, and a masters in family counseling. For the last nine years, she has managed laboratories for two professors at the Massachusetts Institute of Technology.

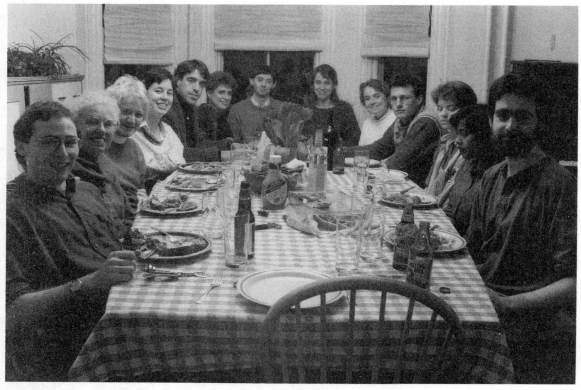

"Dinner with Friends." The Wendell Street Cooperative House, Cambridge, Massachusetts. Photographer: Daniel Labovitz.

BETTY DEXTER

I'm an only child, my parents are dead, I'm divorced, and my children are launched and live all over the country. I have no particular group of people to help me define where I'm going to live. Perhaps the depth of your relationship with your nuclear family is what dictates your need for community living—I feel it has for me. It's a lot easier for me to move than it is for people with lots of family ties, but because of that, I really have to step out more to look for an interesting social life.

I've had years and years of experience living in community. It all began after my divorce, when I rented out rooms in our home just to keep my family afloat. After a while, we wanted to leave the area. My children and I took a house-building course in Maine, and together we built our own low-cost home in the woods. But Maine does not have many high-paying jobs, so when my last son left home, I decided to find a community situation near Boston. For the first few months, this meant living in a boardinghouse, with few connections among the "roomies."

An Intergenerational Community

Every day I searched the personal ads for openings in cooperative homes in the area, and I finally found one for a sixteen-room, intergenerational community established by a trust some thirty years ago. I called immediately and was interviewed by phone. This was followed by an invitation to dinner to meet the whole "family"—and finally, much to my delight, I was accepted into the community.

There are twelve of us living here, ranging in age from twenty-two to sixty-two, sharing meals, chores, responsibilities, and fun. Our ad says that we don't allow pets or smoking and are for the most part vegetarian. We emphasize our age spread and say up front that we value diversity. We welcome people from other cultures and ethnic groups. However, the one diversity we are not looking for is political; many of us would find it difficult to live with right-wing people.

We each cook our own breakfast and lunch—and agree to shop, cook, and clean for community dinners twice a month. I think it's great to have twenty-two evenings when I can come home, put my feet up, and wait for dinner to be served. We rotate general shopping (two people do it every six weeks) and divide up the chores of daily living, like paying bills, collecting rent, and cleaning common areas. You can always ask for a change of job or swap with someone. Nobody ends up doing the same old job for a lifetime. We meet twice a month for decision-making sessions, and have communal dinners at least three nights a week. People are asked to make at least a one-year commitment to the house.

Unlike many single people my age, I don't have to worry about repairing, furnishing, painting, or insuring a house. And the diversity is so stimulating. In our home we have music and art lovers, joggers, sports fans, avid readers, and theater buffs like me. A couple of times, all of us have vacationed together at a lovely lodge in Vermont, where we spent our time enjoying one another's company in new ways, swimming, dancing, and playing ball. Some of us enjoy flowers and go to the flower shows; some enjoy movies and go off in small groups to see the latest ones. We celebrate many holidays together—everyone's birthdays, Christmas, Chanukah, and Thanksgiving.

This sunny kitchen, dining room, and living room are considered common spaces. Most of us have family or friends sleep over a couple of times a year, and there are guest rooms for them. Once a year we have a painting party for the common rooms, with lots of food and laughter. Each of us decorates and cleans our own private space. I've been here the longest and therefore have the largest apartment (two-and-a-half rooms) filled with furniture from home, plants, my treasured books and paintings. My rent is three hundred and sixty-eight dollars a month, including food, phone, utilities—everything.

My weekends are full. Since I discovered the Elderhostel program of weeklong vacations on college campuses around the world, I've spent weeks in several states and Nova Scotia and plan a trip to China soon. I attend a local ashram for yoga exercises and some of my meals. One of my major activities is hiking on weekends with the Appalachian Mountain Club.

We All Like a Clean Home

We're just like any other family who needs to share time and daily lives. And our home is like any other home of people who want to live well. We all like a clean home—enjoy moments of solitude—and the opportunity to share our days with caring others.

Living here has its joys and its problems, like in any other "family." One of the most difficult things for me is having to constantly break in new people. The average stay here is two years, so there is a fair amount of turnover. The phone rings all day after we advertise. We have to explain our life-style over and over again.

People share concerns about what would happen if they became ill. My experience has been good. I had a bad back a few weeks ago, and my housemates were very supportive and helpful. One of the original "family" members was cared for here until she was ninety-one years old. Arrangements were made for her to go to a local nursing home when she became deaf and blind, and there she lived to be one hundred years old.

In this house we have had some trouble with older males who have not carried their weight—who have expected to be cared for by the women of the house. One even asked an outside woman friend to cook for him whenever it was his turn. We finally had to ask him to leave, but that's delicate and difficult. We haven't really worked out a good way to do it.

Recently there has been some tension in the house. We've hired a professional social worker to come interview each member of the house, and try to elicit things that seem too sensitive for house meetings. That seems like a good investment.

For me, group living is providing companionship, good living, and fun—far outweighing any of the alternatives. I wouldn't even consider living alone. I see myself in the future becoming a passionate spokesperson, helping people of all ages find community wherever they live.

Church-Initiated Intergenerational Living: The Virginia Robinson House

This fifth type of small-group living was developed by the ministers of six United Churches of Christ in Newton, Massachusetts, who perceived the need for housing alternatives for semi-independent elders. To meet this need, funds were gathered from a bank mortgage, private foundations, church loans, gifts, and two federal grants. In 1982, the Virginia Robinson House (named for its founder), originally a private single-family dwelling, was purchased for $150,000. The ten residents of the lovely Queen Anne Victorian house, which is within easy walking distance of shopping, banks, a post office, library, senior center, and transportation, range in age from seven to ninety-four. They enjoy their own private bed-sitting room (three are large enough for couples), parking space for six, and a sizable garden space. The residents prepare their own meals but eat together at least once a week, and they hold weekly house meetings with a trained facilitator.

Today, this house is a happy, intergenerational home of venturesome people who share decisions on how their home will be run, chores, and a common space.

* * *

Small-group living is just one in a broad spectrum of community-housing alternatives. For many people in their middle and later years, it is a personal choice, not a last-resort option.

Shared living may not solve all of your problems, but it is very likely to meet many of your needs. You do not have to make a lifetime commitment to anyone sharing the arrangement, as you do in a family. Whether you live there for one year or several, it may be the perfect answer in a period of crisis or transition in your life.

There is no question that shared living helps those struggling with insufficient incomes. It is the least expensive (and easiest to implement) form of community living, offering a pleasant environment at a low rent. It is a more economical way for people of all ages to achieve a quality life-style. But, perhaps most important of all, small-group living arrangements provide others to talk to at the end of a day, to be available to you in times of joy or sorrow, and to offer the companionship so often missing in the lives of people as they age.

The shared housing movement in the United States has been local and small scale, primarily supported by private funding.

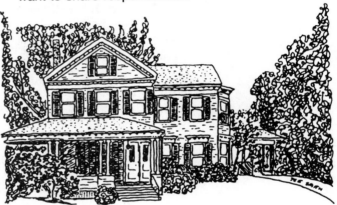
The Virginia Robinson House, Newtonville, Massachusetts.

If it is to spread, more governmental and/or religious organizational support will be needed. Rigid zoning laws (formed to protect the fading nuclear family life-style) need to be challenged—not in each local community but nationally.

Small-group homes rooted in the community are certainly one part of the solution to both the housing crisis in this country and to the growing isolation and loneliness of so many Americans of all ages. Living with a group of people can be a challenging and exciting experience for anyone. If you feel that it might be right for you, consider the following questions:

1. *Would it be better for me to share my home or to become a home sharer in another house?* People report that it is often difficult to move into an already established home of one of the members.

2. *How much rent will I be able to pay?*

3. *How many people will I feel comfortable living with?* Very small groups may be vulnerable to strong personalities or relationships that are too intense. They are also more concerned about an illness of one of the members and vacancies.

   Groups of six to fifteen provide enough people from which to choose friends and a larger group to contribute to the total housing costs, skill sharing, and work force.

4. *Should I look for an "extended family," a friendly but separate relationship within my new home, or a tenant/landlord relationship?*

5. *How will I find like-minded people with compatible needs?* Each person deciding to investigate small-group living possibilities should question whether they want to live with peers and/or young people, with their own sex or both women and men, single people or couples, people currently working or retirees.

   Ask yourself how important cleanliness is in your life. Can you tolerate clutter? Does noise disturb you? How do you feel about pets? smoking? alcohol use?

   If possible, have a trial living period of a week or more.

6. *Where would I like to live?* Location is very important. Accessibility to stores, transportation, health services, cultural and educational events may be even more important than whether you live in a city or in the country.

   Also, do you want to live near your immediate family, relatives, or friends?

7. **Will I still be driving my own car?** This is necessary in many communities located in suburban or rural areas.

8. **How much private space will I need?** A room of one's own is essential for solitude, a base of operations, and a retreat from the stimulation, expectations, and natural tensions of group living.

    You should also consider whether you need a private bathroom, space to entertain visitors privately (but not in the bedroom), professional work space, and parking or garage space.

9. **How do I learn to share space and work responsibilities with non-relatives?** When residents contribute personal possessions for use in shared space, it supports a sense of belonging. Sharing of household chores, planning and decision making help people feel they are a necessary part of the group.

    Remember that it takes time to form the camaraderie you may be looking for.

10. **How will decisions about daily life be made?** Form preliminary, flexible guidelines with all concerned. Be creative. There are no binding rules. You can change them as you go along.

    Guidelines will need to include use of common space, meals to be shared, the distribution of shopping and clean-up chores, the importance of cleanliness, a guest policy, and methods for handling the illness of a member.

    Whenever possible, make decisions by consensus. Provide time at least once a month for house meetings.

    Plan in the beginning how the group will handle a housemate who doesn't fit in after a few months. Develop guidelines for choosing a new person.

Chapter Three

Women's Search for Housing

Housing is a critical issue for midlife and older women. Although this book is written for people over forty, for women and for men, for those married and for those who are single, sheer statistics mandate that women especially need to think about and plan their future living arrangements.

In the United States, home ownership is a cherished goal, and 64 percent of Americans have achieved it. Why then is home ownership an unrealized dream for many women? For elderly single women over sixty-five and for women who maintain families with children, finding decent, affordable housing is one of their greatest difficulties. And yet, where we live and how we live is an intrinsic part of our daily existence. Finding an affordable home that meets our needs may be one of the key challenges women face in the second half of life.

It is no secret that American women live, on average, seven years longer than men. Women have a statistically higher chance of spending a number of years alone at the end of their lives, and as a result, older women are the fastest-growing singles group in America. Consider these numbers:

- There are 146 older women for every 100 older men. This sex ratio increases with age to a high of 256 women for each 100 men, for persons 85 and older.

- Older men are twice as likely to be married as are older women—78 percent of men as compared with 41 percent of women.

- Half of all older women are widows. There are five times as many widows as widowers.

- 82 percent of older men live in family settings, as compared to 57 percent of older women.

- Nearly seven million elderly women live alone; they outnumber elderly men who live alone by nearly four to one.

(Source: A *Profile of Older Americans 1989*, AARP).

In 1900, life expectancy was about forty-eight years for women; today it is almost eighty-two—an increase of thirty-four years in less than one century. This longevity is unprecedented in the history of humankind.

The extension of life expectancy and the longevity gap have combined to produce very unfortunate social and economic consequences for women now in their older years of life. Housing problems are closely linked to low income and high poverty rates. According to U.S. government statistics analyzed in 1989 by the Women's Research and Education Institute, a high percentage of the elderly poor are female. Older women have a median income of $6,734 a year and a poverty rate of 15 percent, compared to 8 percent for older men.

Even among older female homeowners, the median income was a low $8,254. Among renters, the median income for single older women drops as low as $5,000 a year, a staggering figure considering that more than half of all women householders are renters. Renters of all ages pay a higher percentage of income for housing than owners. Women renters are far more likely to pay a large percentage of their income for housing and to be vulnerable to forces they cannot control, such as rising rents and displacement. The problem is most severe for black and Hispanic women. They are more likely to be renters, very poor, and living in substandard housing.

Many midlife women with children are female heads of households, but there is a growing shortage of housing that they can afford. Many must "double up" temporarily with relatives or friends. Today women are beginning to realize that they have a growing number of life-style choices, and that it is never too soon to plan for the second half of their lives. The middle years can be a time to explore new ways of living that will enhance all of the later years. Residing with women of the same age or in a mixed-age women's community is likely to become the first choice for a growing number of women.

Is Housing a Major Concern for Middle-class Women?

This is a question the Older Women's League (OWL) of Manhattan sought to answer. How did their members feel about where and with whom they would live as older women? OWL called a special meeting on housing and invited me to share some of the research I had gathered for this book. They warned that only a handful of women might show up, but the number of attendees surprised us all. These women were *very* concerned about what the future held for them. One woman expressed her fears poignantly: "With the clear perception of a fifty-seven-year-old, I see nothing to prevent me from being poor when I have to stop work. I feel squeezed into the neck of a timer, scrambling frantically to prevent the sand from engulfing me. Housing in my later years is my biggest concern!"

A small survey of the group revealed an average yearly income of $32,000—ranging from $12,000 for a single seventy-year-old woman to a combined income of $50,000 for a fifty-nine-year-old married woman. These women had begun to think about the issues of future housing as they approached the age of sixty, or became widowed or divorced. Many felt forced to make immediate changes in their life-styles because of exorbitant rent increases, a need for companionship, and deteriorating neighborhoods. And they all spoke about their need for privacy and autonomy, but agreed that these could be achieved in intergenerational communities with compatible people. They were women ready for change.

Women's Housing: From Dreams to Reality

The Dreaming

I believe that if you can fantasize your future, your dreams can become a reality. I asked the women of Manhattan OWL to fantasize

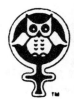 # Older Women's League

GREATER NEW YORK CHAPTER

INVITES YOU TO EXPLORE

HOUSING OPTIONS FOR OLDER WOMEN

Saturday–May 20, 1989
9:30 am to 2:00 pm
H. R. A.–109 East 16th Street
Coffee–Tea–Juice will be served
Lunch Break–Brown-bag it or nearby restaurants

WHERE WILL YOU BE LIVING 5 YEARS FROM NOW???
Plan Ahead. . . . Take Control of Your Life. . . .

So That The Choice Will Be Yours:

[A] Independent, But—
needing help with some
daily living tasks.

[D] Shared Housing—
One or more non-family
members living
together.

[B] Feminist Model—
Affordable, Mixed
Ethnic, Inter-
generational.

[E] Retirement
Communities—
Recreation, Social,
Educational, Health &
Fitness Amenities.

[C] Funding Sources—
Public & Private
Initiatives, Land Trusts,
Nehemiah.

[F] Senior Housing—
Optional Services,
Meals, Recreation,
Housekeeping, etc.

Announcement about exploring housing options sponsored by the Older
Women's League, Greater New York Chapter.

the type of housing they would like for themselves if money were no obstacle. These are their responses:

Dream housing for me would be either a large old Victorian-type house renovated to provide small apartments with private baths, or a compoundlike series of small homes with a communal garden, library, and social room. One, two, or three women could share each house and pool transportation.

◆ ◆ ◆

I am looking for women who would be willing to start the search for shared housing on an equal footing; women who are intelligent and committed to the idea.

◆ ◆ ◆

I would like to share a house with my dearest friend and perhaps one other person. Ours would be a most interesting ecumenical household with plenty of lively conversation on current events. My friend and I do not always see eye to eye, but our differing views are as stimulating as our shared opinions.

◆ ◆ ◆

I am looking for intellectually stimulating events, an opportunity to share life with others of a similar bent, and to make friends. Nothing gets in my way in thinking about the future except lack of knowledge about what options are available. I'm looking forward to your book so I can be better informed.

◆ ◆ ◆

I would like to sell my small house and build a cottage on my daughter's property in Berkeley, California. I want to be near my family and grandchildren.

◆ ◆ ◆

It would be fun to exchange apartments or living accommodations with someone in whom I have complete confidence. I would like to live a different life-style for two or three months every year.

◆ ◆ ◆

If I have permission to dream, I'll take a home near a lake in a peaceful area of Connecticut—and have a chauffeur drive me into New York City at least two nights a week. I'd like an opportunity to make new friends, develop new interests, and to travel.

◆　◆　◆

I'm really interested in discovering how people accommodate creatively in a group-living situation, so that the group can develop, grow, and serve one another with comfort, ease and love.

Do the people who lived in communal situations in their youth ever dream about community for their later years? Forty-eight-year-old Alice Radosh, who has her Ph.D. in neuropsychology, says, resoundingly, "Yes!"

ALICE RADOSH

My husband and I really loved living collectively in one house with two other couples when our kids were growing up—and I know I will want to do it again later in my life. When we moved out, we moved directly across the street and continued sharing meals and child care for many years. Still no birthday goes by without all of us gathering. There is an understanding that we will share events and some time together on all the holidays.

My kids are gone now; it's just my husband and me. Neither of us want to live in community during this time in our lives. We spent so many years organizing around the needs of kids, that now we're reveling in making plans only for ourselves.

But I do sometimes think about the time twenty-two years from now when I will be seventy. I don't agonize about it, because I believe that community-living arrangements don't necessarily have to be planned far ahead of time. The first time around, if I'd waited until all the pieces seemed right, as many people do, I would probably never have done it.

Is "uncoupling" the time you look for community living, or is it a health crisis, or is it economics? It's clear that I will likely be in a female society in my later years. I've been involved with women's groups all of my life, and the thought of living collectively with women sounds just fine to me.

I feel my options are many. One of the women in the house across the street and I are very sure that eventually we will live together again. We each foresee holding on to the homes we own, in this lovely area of Brooklyn, where we've lived for eighteen years. We know we can live together and we both feel very comfortable here.

My sister lives with her family in California, and every time I see her she says, "We're going to live together when we're older, right?" We share a history, and she would be comfortable to live with. I spend summers with my brother and sister-in-law and could imagine us living together in the future. But I know that not everyone will be in the same place at the same time; some will be ready and others won't. People's schedules and needs don't always coincide.

I think all of these new ways of thinking have to do with the feminist movement, which freed us from the rigidity of nuclear-family living as the only option for life.

Planning Ahead

Tish Sommers, the founder of the National Older Women's League (OWL), shared her dream with other women about a creative alternative to a nursing home. They would call their live-in community the "Last Perch," fill it with compatible women—some ambulatory and others not—all living out their last days in a joyous, beautiful setting. Tish's vision would encourage women to be able to control their own lives to the end.

The Clovers' Retirement Community

Living with life-committed women friends is an old-age alternative. One group of women in their forties began to plan their "Clovers' Retirement Community." These women met at Pennsylvania State University and were part of a peer-counseling group. Ten years later, they were living all over the place (from Boston to Vancouver, British Columbia), were all in primary relationships, and had four children between them. Despite the passing of time, their friendship remained intact, but each of them realized that they missed the kind of nurturing community they had experienced at college.

Over the years, amidst much seriousness and joking, the goal of living together in their old age began to take form. They agreed to meet together once a year for a long weekend and to begin actively planning their later years. Each contributes one hundred dollars a year to a retirement-home fund and has made a commitment to support the others in joy and in sorrow, throughout their lives. They visit or phone whenever possible, send little notes or gifts for no reason at all, have a twice yearly newsletter ("The Clover Chronicle"), a round-robin letter, and a Clovers' photo album. The knowledge of life commitment ("these people are there for me until we die, no matter what I do or what I become") has led to intense, open, and trusting relationships. As they became friends with primary partners, children, and parents of other Clovers, they began to envision the possibility of an earlier intergenerational community. As one of the Clovers, Kathy McGuire, says, "Having Clovers' retirement to look forward to leads me to take better care of my health than ever before. I have no intention of missing all the fun, and surprisingly enough, I can hardly wait to grow old!"

This simple plan is one any group of friends could adopt. The response of other women I meet as I lecture around the country to the Clovers' ideas has been very enthusiastic. Many of them have said that such a fantasy has always been in the back of their minds, but they never dreamed it could become a reality.

Not content to wait for the government to act on the housing crisis, many small groups are forging unique solutions to their housing and social needs. An excellent example of a well-organized housing action comes from housing consultant Jean Mason, a sixty-five-year-old psychologist. For more than two years she has been searching for community living for herself and her husband—and assisting others to find a creative housing solution to their needs. Jean conducts workshops and seminars on shared-housing alternatives as a part of the program "Midlife Options for Women," in Brookline, Massachusetts. I drove up to Boston to interview her.

JEAN MASON

I've been interested in housing for a very long time. Even when we had young children, I thought how ridiculous it was to feel so alone and isolated. Why couldn't we share lives—and possessions like washing machines, garden equipment, and such? I've come to the obvious conclusion that isolation is at the heart of much of the depression women feel—and that much effort should be made to combat this on the level of the built environment.

The group planning I do with women begins with our Saturday workshops, which introduce interested people to the wide range of housing alternatives. I believe that people, once organized, can do it for themselves. In one group, sixteen women have been meeting regularly. They are all working professionals between the ages of thirty-five and sixty-five; they are all single, have adult children, and own their own homes. As they have come to know and trust one another, some are moving on to the next step—looking for a joint-home purchase or rental together. They feel that the co-op ideas work best, with each person buying their own unit, having a share of the common space, and controlling the selection of housemates.

Among the problems that have surfaced are the high cost of land and housing, the rigid zoning regulations, and the lack of any really good models of shared housing to examine. This is where your book should be very helpful.

On the personal side, my husband and I would like to share housing with other like-minded couples. Several months ago we were able to interest a local private developer in our ideas. He was about to break ground on a traditional co-op, which would open in about a year. We put an ad in a Harvard magazine asking for "independent professional people interested in discussing shared living arrangements." To our surprise, twenty-four people of different ages came forward. All were homeowners and wanted to explore the next step in their lives.

But, in the long run, we would have had to move too fast to sell our own homes and to buy into the co-op in a year's time. Although everyone expressed a concern about not wanting to live alone if/when their spouses died, the crisis was not yet present. Everyone needed time to get used to the idea of making such a major change in their living arrangements, and perhaps some of them will be ready at a later date. The seeds of community living were planted.

We all learned from this experience and are much wiser now. We know that good preparation and timing are essential.

Thinking About a Shared Future

Martha Tabor worked with me in the initial stages of this book, contributing her excellent photography. She was personally interested in the search for a small community. She says:

I'm a forty-eight-year-old woman—a free-lance graphic artist and photographer. I have been living alone or in intergenerational communal households in Washington, D.C., since my divorce many years ago. Now I'm exploring the possibilities of buying and sharing a home with two of my close friends from a feminist theology group. Both women are about my age, are divorced, and have grown children. One works for the government, and the other is a free-lance musician. None of us lives with the fantasy that Mr. Right will come along or that we should wait for him. That's not a future worth waiting for. The prospect of sharing a home with friends is exciting and scary at the same time. We've asked the marriage and family relations committee of our Quaker Fellowship to help us in the process.

Widows Who Don't Want to Live with Adult Children

One of my students at New York University told the class the following story about her mother:

The shock of my father's death and her total dependence on him left my mother in a miserable state. She suffered medical problems for five years and finally moved in with my older sister. She would stay several months with one of us, temporarily creating turmoil in each household.

Three years ago, she and a group of long-term friends—widows living with adult children in the suburbs—decided to live independently. They have their name on an apartment waiting list in Chinatown and are excitedly planning to share their lives. My mother is again the vital, strong woman she once was.

Searching for a Women's Community

Two women in their sixties have joined forces in their search for people interested in creating a small women's communal house. They have been friends for years; back in the seventies, they began thinking about developing a community with a social-change focus.

Both divorced, they have found themselves on the move. One woman was evicted from a home she shared with her mother in Brooklyn, because they had no tenant's rights. Both are struggling financially and cannot afford to pay the rent on a city apartment.

They describe their situations with the words "nomad," "gypsy," "wanderer," and "homeless." They have shared various types of apartments with acquaintances or have relied on the largess of their friends. Neither wants to depend on adult children, although realistically they know they won't be left to live on the streets or to starve. As one says, "My worst scenario is being a burden, having to live with my children."

They would like to have a home to spend their remaining years in. For them, community living can make that possible.

Three Women and Their "Geriatric Commune"

When I mentioned my upcoming book while staying in a little town in Massachusetts, a minister there said, "Oh, you *must* see Lucy Conant." The hours spent with Lucy that day and on future occasions were among the most delightful of all my interviewing. Her unusual background, as well as her exciting plans for the future, are an integral part of this book.

Lucy Conant is a sixty-one-year-old single public-health nurse with a doctoral degree in sociology. She was the dean of nursing at the University of North Carolina for seven years, until she decided to take early retirement to fulfill another dream.

Brought up by a professional family who lived on a farm, Lucy bought a farm of her own in the small village of Chester, Massachusetts. After retirement, she settled into farming an acre of land, raising and showing a special breed of sheep, and participating in community activities. She loved her new life-style.

But ten years later she began to think ahead to the future.

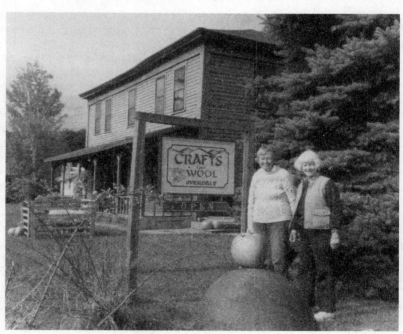

Lucy Conant and Virginia Brown, co-owners of "The Old House" in Chester, Massachusetts.

LUCY CONANT

One's early sixties seems like a good time to think about and plan for old age. My health is good, but I'm increasingly aware that in the not-too-distant future, all of this farm work will get to be too much.

I began to talk to two other single women friends, classmates at Yale, about living close to one another in our later years. One of these women was keenly interested. She has no family at all and plans to retire soon from her position as director of a large nursing-home facility in New York City.

The second woman has an extended family of nieces and nephews, as I do, and plans to continue directing her home health agency for several more years. But she was interested for the future. Both women have been involved in nursing homes, and they know they never want to live in one. Me either. My plan was to live in the middle of a small village where I could watch the kids go by every day.

Just last year I saw two wonderful, older widowed men-friends in our village begin to deteriorate and end up in a nursing home. They would have been less lonely and bewildered if they had planned a few years earlier to combine forces by purchasing either an apartment of their own or joining a retirement community.

Last year, a big house on the main road of the village was put on the market. This was the opportunity we had been waiting for. It had originally been a tavern, with a good-size kitchen, four big rooms downstairs, and five very large rooms upstairs. It is within walking distance of the village.

And so, stage one of our plan began. We purchased the house and rented out the back part to a young family. We laughingly refer to it as our "geriatric commune of the future." We orga-nized a weekend craft shop for women in the village, which was located in our front parlor. Zoning laws are a potential problem, but we figure that when we are ready to move in, we will be able to present a good hardship-and-need case to the town board and get a variance.

One friend wants to retire in two years, and so we have got-ten serious about our plan. She loves to fix up old houses—but I must admit that painting and scraping are not exactly my cup of tea. So, for stage two, we have contracted out some of the reno-vating work. Our plan is to build at least four apartments right away, each with their own private bedroom, bath, and small kitchen. I insisted on a kitchen of my own so that when I wake up early in the morning, I can get breakfast and just putter around. We'll have dinner together every evening and maybe some lunches. Whoever has the best legs will live upstairs, and we may eventually have to install one of those seats that takes you up and down the stairs.

We have other classmates and a network of friends who are amused but interested in our ideas for themselves. We do a lot of joking about it, because when you think of a commune, you think of hippies—not a bunch of old ladies. My family thinks this is a great idea. My nephew said to his father, "Thank God she'll be able to look after herself." I think families are relieved when we take over the planning of our future.

In our new home, each of us will have enough space to do our own thing, and yet we will be together so we can keep an eye out for one another. We'll be as independent as we want to be. We laugh as we figure out that one of us might have problems with their head and someone else with their eyes or legs, but we plan to put it all together, and add up to one able-bodied person.

This is a copy of a letter Lucy Conant sent to her classmates at the Yale School of Nursing. She said their fortieth reunion would take place this summer.

A NEW FORM OF RECYCLING
FOR FUN AND FRIENDSHIP

Dear classmates of the 1950 Yale School of Nursing:

Have you thought about the advantages of village living in your retirement years? If so, consider the possibilities in Chester, Massachusetts, listed on the National Historic Register and located between the Connecticut River and the Berkshire hills.

How about inexpensive, independent housing with your former classmates nearby—with whom to play—and who will water your plants and take care of your cat when you want to travel. Then as we all get older, there will be a familiar support group of old-time friends when and if needed, or desired. Other advantages to consider:

- The cost of living is lower than in cities and resort areas.

- Friendly and competent service people are available, such as handyman, garage mechanic, and household help.

- Excellent health care facilities are just nine miles down the road. Comprehensive care at the Huntington Health Center is provided by a well-established, nonprofit organization. The medical director, by the way, is a former Yale Medical School faculty member.

- Cultural activities of all sorts are within a 30-mile area, including: Williams College, the University of Massachusetts, Smith College, and others. Small city and urban facilities and activities are conveniently located in nearby Westfield and Springfield—plus the world-famous Tanglewood Concerts and Jacob's Pillow Dance Festival.

- The area is abundantly supplied with hiking, camping, skiing and other outdoor recreation facilities for all ages—a plus for attracting visiting children.

The beachhead has been established by Overdale Associates—Lucy, Jean, and Brownie. If you are interested in seeing for yourself, plan with us to make a trip to Chester after our fortieth reunion. If you have some questions let us know.

See you soon.

Lucy

Disabled Older Women

I read about Lillian Holcomb in a women's publication called *Broomstick.* We have been corresponding ever since about the often invisible group of women who will come of age with a major disability. Where and how will they live in the second half of their lives? This is Lillian's concern on both a personal and a professional level.

LILLIAN HOLCOMB

I am a psychologist in my midforties—a minority woman legally blind since birth. Because of several new disabilities resulting from a car crash, I find myself among the present generation of aging disabled women who, for the first time in history, will make it intact to old age—in extreme poverty and isolation. Medical technology has kept us alive, but very little thought has been given to the quality of our lives as we age. Many of us— never "wanted" in marriage and never "wanted" on the career and employment lines—approach old age with nothing to support us except welfare and social security and with no confidence that the government will house us.

To address some of these issues, I have founded DAWS (Differently Abled Women's Support) and a task force in the Seattle, Washington, Older Women's League (OWL).

Several members are exploring the concept of a self-sustaining community where our needs could be addressed by other older professional women. So many aging disabled women are maintaining themselves in their apartments without any help. Mine is a cross between a university professor's office and a gymnasium. I have a treadmill and bike to maintain my pain program. Because of my blindness, I have all manner of nontraditional furniture.

In my seventies I would like to see myself living in an environment that meets my needs for a spiritual, feminist community with an egalitarian philosophy. Together, we would gather the technology for rehabilitation and treatment of chronic pain syndromes that may occur in our aging process. We are pioneers forging new territory, and our lives will be most adventuresome, to say the least.

(Interested readers can contact Dr. Holcomb at 1011 Boren Avenue, #114, Seattle, Washington 98104.)

Making Small-Group Housing a Reality

For two years I have been interviewing women around the country who are living in communities they created for themselves and others. Many of these women dreamed of one day living in an urban center in their middle and later years. Elizabeth Freeman has succeeded in forming The Molly Hare cooperative house in Durham, North Carolina.

Elizabeth (whom I mentioned briefly in chapter 1) spent years educating women about alternative housing options in her role as president of the Durham Older Women's League. She received a grant to run a workshop entitled "What's Down the Road? Housing Alternatives for Older Women." This meeting generated so much excitement that a housing task force was formed, assisted by an architect and the Durham Center for Community Self-Help. Their original plans to build a fourteen-unit, single-story apartment building in downtown Durham fell through. But as Elizabeth says, she "dove in" to work on plan two.

ELIZABETH FREEMAN

At that point I discovered an existing apartment building that seemed ideal for cooperative living. It had six units on a quiet street near Duke University and was within walking distance of shops and services.

Through the Durham Center, I got the financial, legal, and business help I needed to purchase the building for $170,000 and *set up a cooperative. I worked with the center to design financial arrangements that would appeal to older women. We decided on a $7,000 to $9,000 down payment for buying into the co-op—an affordable, limited equity—plus monthly fees.*

We developed promotional materials and received good local publicity, because The Molly Hare Cooperative is Durham's first. We stressed the advantages of co-op living for older women: You own your own unit; you can decide who lives with you; it is safe and affordable and will remain so for years to come; it can't go condo; you hold lifelong occupancy rights; you get your money back if you decide to leave; you can will your share; as an owner, you can take the mortgage interest and taxes as an income-tax deduction.

It always takes longer than expected to complete a project like this. However, the three years didn't seem too long, particularly when the gradual and steady growth yielded such rewards as companionship, a caring environment, financial stability, and the sure knowledge that what I was doing was a model for others.

The Molly Hare Cooperative is a place for neighbors and friends to live together, building a community within their living space. The six lovely modern apartments are energy efficient and include modern appliances and hardwood floors. Occupancy fees depend on the size and condition of the apartment selected, and they range from $400 to $572 a month. Tax deductions reduce these fees by $50 to $120, depending upon an individual's tax bracket. These monthly fees include principal and interest on the mortgage, property taxes, insurance, occasional repairs, and some utilities. Members have established a future capital improvements reserve fund. Elizabeth continues:

It became obvious early on that a most important task was to keep the apartments rented, because the mortgage had to be paid. This meant that as soon as a renter who was still in the apartment (and not interested in joining) left, the primary consideration was to get someone in as soon as possible. Fortunately, the first vacancies were filled by two individuals who were attracted to cooperative living. There were now three of us.

These renters, aware of the advantages of this type of living, began a policy of "renting to buy." Although pushed by financial considerations, this proved to be a good idea both for the renter and the co-op. It provided an interval of time to make sure there was a match between the individual and the group.

At this point we are about to have a full complement of members. The last renter will move in in a few months, leaving us with just one opening. As we are now well known in the community as a thriving housing cooperative, there are several persons interested in joining. A committee will decide who it will be.

We have attracted women of varying ages, and it has become obvious to me that this has many advantages. The two graduate students gave us energy and enthusiasm—and we, I feel sure, showed them the joys and wisdom accompanying the process of growing old. The age of members ranges from forty-four (a woman disabled by an auto accident and much in need of the kind of protective and nurturing environment we provide), to a seventy-six-year-old retired homemaker, and include a sociologist (fifty-seven), a retired professor (sixty-nine), and a retired counselor (seventy).

We believe our persistence is already paying off. One woman in town is considering converting her four-apartment building into a co-op. Though ours is small in size, it acts as a model for others seeking to meet similar needs. I am briefing local real-estate agents about the cooperative-housing concept. They are enthusiastic, because it provides a real answer to older women facing the question: "Sell my home? Then what?"

(Interested readers can contact The Molly Hare Cooperative in care of Elizabeth Freeman, 209 Watts Street, Durham, North Carolina 27701.)

Phoenix House: A Women's Place

Located on the outer fringe of a university neighborhood in a racially and economically mixed area of Philadelphia, Phoenix House has been a haven for a diverse group of women, ranging in age from twenty-four to sixty-one, since 1977. A unique characteristic of this particular community is its success in terms of caring for the financial needs of women in their middle years and beyond.

It is important for many women, as they enter their middle years, to own the house in which they live. Phoenix House is an excellent model for how this can be accomplished if women live as part of a group. For example, members estimate that women can earn less than ten thousand dollars a year and still afford to

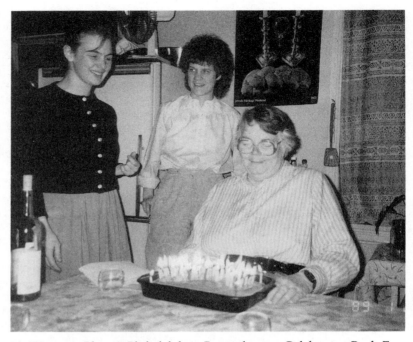

"A Women's Place," Philadelphia, Pennsylvania. Celebrating Ruth Fansler's birthday are (left to right) Hanne Weedon, Gretchen Boise, and Ruth Fansler.

live in Phoenix House. (The land for the house is owned by a nonprofit corporation, the Life Center Association, a land trust, which leases the land to users with the expectation of maintaining, preserving, and enhancing its long-range resource values.) Individual payments for group members are $147 per month, which includes the monthly mortgage, insurance, maintenance, and basic telephone and utilities payments. Each woman puts eighteen dollars per week into a "kitty" for food and supplies purchased at local food co-ops. All repairs and maintenance costs are shared.

Florence Rosoff, the founder, writes: "When I was fifty-seven I started dreaming about a women's house. I knew I would enjoy living with women of different ages, sexual preferences, classes, races, ethnic and religious backgrounds. I like differences; I like the creative conflict that results from living in a pluralistic house."

HOUSEMATES WANTED

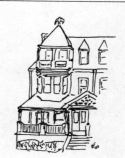

FOR
WOMEN'S COMMUNAL HOUSEHOLD

WE ARE
—a supportive feminist community, in existence for over ten years
—diverse in age, nationality, background, and sexual orientation
—non-smoking, and mostly vegetarian
—part of a cooperatively owned land trust, with six cooperatively managed buildings
—located in a spacious charming house in West Philadelphia

—*seeking friendly reliable women who want to share the advantages and responsibilities of cooperative living.*

We share meals, chores, and house repairs.

Expenses range from $165–190 per month for rent and utilities. Food is about $20 per week.
CALL 724-5142

P.S. WE HAVE a dog and two cats (no more pets, please).

A flyer designed to attract potential housemates.

At the time of my visit, I interviewed two women over forty who characterize this diversity. Ruth Fansler, sixty-one, has been divorced for many years and is the mother of two adult sons. She has a masters degree in math and now works in an administrative capacity for a Quaker organization called Friends World Committee. She earns less than twenty thousand dollars a year, but has fully paid health insurance. In terms of savings or pension, she has very little. Ruth chose an all-women's house because, "I've been divorced now as long as I was married. When I moved here, I had just come out of a relationship and felt like I wanted to be with women. I feel more comfortable and relaxed around women. Here I can just be myself."

Joan Mikelsky, forty-three, has never married and considers herself a social-change activist. She has a masters degree in early childhood education but has been working as a technical editor for an educational researcher at Temple University. She is also president of the Women's Alliance for Job Equity, which deals with working women's issues, middle-aged women in the work force, and job discrimination. She makes a little more than twenty thousand dollars a year, which is the most she has ever earned. Her job includes a good benefits and pension plan, and Joan has started an IRA for the future.

I asked Joan how she felt about her all-female living situation. She replied, "Living here has taught me how to really enjoy the company of women. This life-style has helped me to explore my femininity."

(Interested readers can contact Phoenix House in care of The Life Center Association, 4722 Baltimore Avenue, Philadelphia, Pennsylvania 19143.)

Lesbian Women-Centered Communities

At least ten percent of women in the United States are lesbians. Twenty years ago, groups of lesbians around the country became pioneers in creating ways to survive and thrive in a women-centered community. One example of such a community is The Pagoda and Crone's Nest Community in Florida.

In 1984, a group of younger women from the Pagoda Community of St. Augustine, Florida, invited me to be on a national board of consultants for a new project, Creative Retirement Options for Nurturance and Empowerment. They were interested in expanding their small community to an intergenerational one, where they could learn from and honor the lifelong contributions and work of older women. A nearby space, called "Crone's Nest," was to become an alternative-housing arrangement for a group of older women living in isolation or in institutions. Their vision was:

> To create a place that welcomed women, whether physically strong or not, of whatever color, creed, economic condition, or sexual preference; to respect each woman's choice to live as quiet or active a life-style as she desired; to challenge the dominant cultural attitudes on aging and death, and to try to deal openly with fears, beliefs, and expectations of these issues.
>
> To begin with women who are mobile and provide for them when they become less mobile; to emphasize healing, health, and holistic growth on a physical, emotional, mental, and spiritual level; to be knowledgeable about preventive measures, natural health care, and alternatives to drugs; to have a building with an infirmary, so that a woman who comes to live here knows she can stay until the day she dies and not be separated from her friends.

The Pagoda Community is a small seaside community of lesbians. Established in 1973, it contains a cluster of privately owned beach cottages, a pool, and a group-owned cultural center that includes a library, theater, natural-food store, spiritual center, meeting space, kitchen, and guest rooms (for both straight and gay women). Seventeen lesbian women live in the community. The youngest is twenty-six, and seven members are over age fifty. Fiftieth birthdays are the occasion of a special community celebration.

When cottages are available, they rent for about $350 a month. The one-bedroom rustic cottages are furnished, have air-conditioning and heat, a stove and a refrigerator, and are "a one minute walk from the ocean." Cottages, at the moment, are not wheelchair accessible. Although pets are allowed, strict rules exist about their care.

Residents of the Pagoda meet in a group one evening a week to work out interpersonal issues or problems that individuals have not been able to solve by themselves or with the help of a chosen facilitator. The residents are women of diverse spiritual

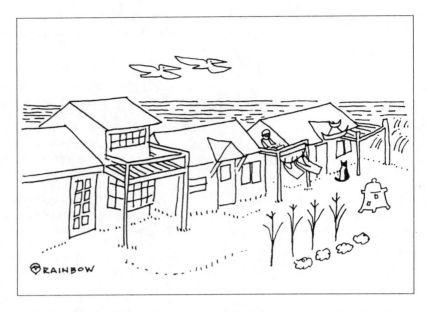

Two sketches by "Rainbow" of the Pagoda Community, St. Augustine, Florida.

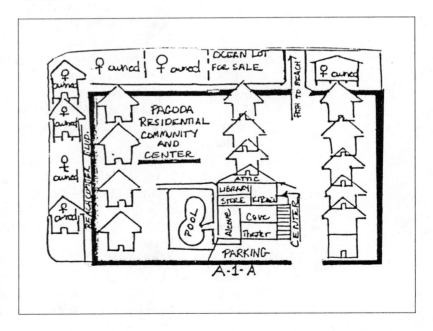

perspectives. At present, no women of color live in the community, but they are welcome.

Pagoda guidelines state:

- We are a relatively quiet and settled community. Although we like to have fun, this is not a partying atmosphere.

- We try to do everything possible to make decisions by consensus.

- We are a developing community and we continually make mistakes. We therefore want women here who are flexible and who can take a joke.

- We strive to be a nonviolent community.

- We have established a trial period of four months for all new residents. If during that time we do not believe that a new woman's residency would be beneficial to her or the community, we reserve the right to ask her to leave. We exercise this right very sparingly and with great respect for its seriousness.

This successful, growing community serves as a model for both straight and gay women who want to create new types of women-centered communities in the future.

(Interested readers can contact The Pagoda and Crone's Nest Community at 207 Coastal Highway, St. Augustine, Florida 32084.)

. . .

I found the best housing resources for older lesbians in a book entitled *Lesbian Land.* The editor, Joyce Cheney, completed a trek around the United States to visit urban and rural lesbian communities established in the seventies. I perused the book for references to women over forty and found these voices of midlife lesbian women:

> We continue to struggle with many familiar issues:
> competition, jealousy, class differences, power dynam-
> ics, and racism. But there are many days of gladness:
> dinner waiting when you come home, a feeling that
> your life does count for something—that you have
> helped create something that is needed.
> Womanshare, Grants Path, Oregon

> Sometimes I don't want to welcome the unending
> stream of visitors. I don't return their excitement at

meeting me, of being here. I just want them to go away and not mess up the kitchen or use my stuff in the bathroom. I am older, but not necessarily wiser. The old ways still take me as they can my younger sisters.

Lavender Hill, Mendocino, California

As the situation of world hunger, thirst, despair, and madness increases, it is apparent to some of us that radical changes in the American way of life are soon to occur. People must find a way out of cities, and for women, especially lesbian women, it is nearly impossible without a lot of resources. We intend to be such a resource—a lifeline.

Greenhope, East Hardwick, Vermont

I'm not going to build my house for ten years. I've got places to go and people to see. But, I'm going to grow old and die here. I've been looking for a home for a long time. I get more of a sense of real community here, more of a sense of family, than from my own family.

Maude's Land, in the Ozarks

Kvindelandet, or the "women's land," in Denmark became a home for women all over the world. Visitors were always welcomed, and they came from many different countries. This unique women's community lasted five years, but was forced to close when an oil corporation set up noisy rigs across the street.

Despite its short existence, however, *Kvindelandet* was not a failure. As one former resident testifies, "I still have not come upon the kind of cooperation and harmony in a living situation that I found on *Kvindelandet.* What do approval and success mean here? To find a center and balance in yourself, to be creative, to work in harmony. This is the mortar of our women's community . . . a good example of how women can create a fascinating, flourishing society."

Women grew from their experiences in group living, and many have founded new communities.

Some of the communities mentioned in *Lesbian Land* were founded by women in their middle years. The founder of

Maude's Land in the Ozarks commented: "I think my own desperation was part of what caused this land to happen. Approaching fifty, I didn't want to spend another ten years trying to make connections. I was going to do it now, or it wasn't ever going to get done."

Another middle-aged woman purchased *two* country spaces, which are open to both lesbian and straight women to do their art work, write, or retreat from daily pressures. Willow, in Napa Valley, California, is home to five women and several pets. Six buildings are on the property, with a main house containing nine bedrooms, five bathrooms, a sauna, and a massage room. Outside is a deck, solar-heated pool, hot tub, tennis court, and vineyard. The Galisteo Inn, in Galisteo, New Mexico, is a large 230-year-old adobe structure with a pool, spa, and sauna. Twenty women can be accommodated. "We want to make this beautiful space, with such pleasant surroundings and facilities, available to many women who would not otherwise be able to afford to stay in a place like the Willow." Other lesbian communities that welcome midlife women include: Arco Iris, in Ponca, Arkansas—a spiritual community for women and children of color; Beechtree, Forest-burgh, New York—space for disabled people to live autonomously; DW Outpost, Ava, Missouri—an artist's community; Greenhope, East Hardwick, Vermont—a holistic healing farm advocating yoga, macrobiotics, physical labor, co-counseling, and spiritual inspiration.

Lesbian Connection, a bimonthly newsletter, published by the Helen Diner Memorial Women's Center (P.O. Box 811, East Lansing, MI 48826), offers current information about lesbian communities that welcome new residents and/or visitors.

Joyce Cheney reports with candor which lesbian communities, created with such hope, have succeeded and which have failed. It is her desire that the success stories will encourage women's visions of living on the land, and that women will learn from the difficulties others have already experienced.

*   *   *

All of the women described in this chapter have been pioneers in creating new types of community life-styles for themselves and for other women. I applaud their efforts. As the number of older women around the country (and around the world) continues to increase at a much greater rate than the number of older men, we will need new housing options to meet their diverse financial, social, and emotional needs. These role models have shown us some ways to do so.

Chapter Four

Cohousing and the American Dream of Community

As we have seen, life-styles have changed dramatically in both Europe and the United States. Now it's time for housing to catch up.

A living arrangement that greatly appeals to my husband and me is one we visited in Sweden. Pioneered in Denmark in 1972, *Bofaellesskab* (literally meaning "living community") is a concept referred to as cohousing in the United States. This housing model can now be found in the Netherlands, Denmark, Sweden, France, Norway, and Germany. It is a novel solution to the isolation felt by individuals and families who live in traditional housing environments, and to the general disappearance of the extended family. This type of housing combines the advantages of yesterday's villages with today's amenities.

Cohousing groups have been successful in Scandinavian countries for two decades, with more than 100 communities established in Denmark. At present, forty-eight separate projects that will house sixteen thousand Danish families are under construction. Many of these are government sponsored and are considered successful alternatives to high-rise public housing.

The Danes say that what they're doing is nothing new. They are creating consciously what used to happen unconsciously before society changed. That was in the days when mothers stayed home, when families lived with or near their relatives, when housing was more affordable, and when families enjoyed a sense of neighborhood.

Cohousing is a grass-roots movement growing out of people's dissatisfaction with existing housing choices. It begins with people whose major bond is the need for affordable housing and a supportive community. But it is primarily the architecture—the unique design of individual homes and shared dwellings—that encourages and even demands a sense of community. The communities are small—between twenty-five and forty clustered homes. Individual houses are designed to be completely self-sufficient. Opportunities for both social interaction and privacy are built in. Front patios face walkways, but bedrooms face private backyards. Cars are parked on the perimeter so that—on the pathways to the houses—children can play safely and adults can socialize with neighbors. Living units are not shared, but virtually everything else is.

In the center of the community is a shared common house. Some communities offer meals there seven nights a week that residents take turns preparing. This makes dinner more convenient and less expensive for those who choose to eat in the common house.

The common house might also be used for meetings, child care, workshops, laundry facilities, guest rooms, or even as a community store. Some have developed miniature office parks, so that people who normally work at home have the best of both worlds. Members share equipment such as lawn mowers and tools, and each household participates in the common chores of everyday life.

Cohousing is a viable option for people who dream of having the privacy of their own home or apartment, as well as the advantages of living in a community. They are people with a wide variety of talents and career goals. They are young and old, married and single. They are willing to work with others, and they believe there is something to be gained from a community where people look out for one another.

Some cohousing projects are newly created, from foundation to finish, in cities or suburbs, whereas others occupy former school buildings, farmhouses, and even factories. Living quarters may be in row houses, town houses, stacked-up apartments, or single-family dwellings. The grounds may be country-spacious or urban-compact. Each community is different—planned for, designed, developed, and managed by the people who make their homes there. Each reflects the different needs for costs, for space, and for recreation. Most are intergenerational—a unique blend of ages, income levels, and unit sizes. Single parents, older people who do not want to live alone, and young families looking for affordable housing are especially interested in the cohousing concept. The residents of each community share a vision of how life should be:

> We've been dreaming about something like this for
> years, but we didn't think it was possible.
> Midlife couple in an American cohousing group

> I don't have to drive to get to my friends: I can walk
> out my door or open my window and they'll be there.
> A divorced woman living alone

> I was not going to just sit in my house alone and get
> older. Here I have complete autonomy and a community just outside my door.
> Retired Danish woman

> It's wonderful to live with people of so many different
> ages and backgrounds.
> Retired Danish man

Bringing the Cohousing Idea to America

Katherine McCamant and her husband, Charles Durrett, both architects, spent more than a year in Denmark researching the cohousing life-style. They created the term *cohousing,* and introduced this community concept to America. Their book *Cohousing: A Contemporary Approach to Housing Ourselves* was published in 1988 by Habitat Press. They believe that cohousing in the United States can be accomplished without government intervention, within the existing framework of legal considerations, financing options, and zoning codes.

With two financial experts, Katherine and Charles have recently formed the CoHousing Development Company. This company will provide services in the areas of group formation and facilitation, site search and acquisition, real-estate brokerage, land development, architectural design, project management, and finance. It works with resident groups throughout the entire development process and provides consulting services nationwide.

Through their workshops and presentations, McCamant and Durrett have facilitated the formation of dozens of cohousing resident groups. Their work has received national recognition including coverage on NBC's "Today Show" and ABC's "World News Tonight." Articles have appeared in *Architecture*, *The Utne Reader*, the *Christian Science Monitor*, the *Los Angeles Times*, and the *Sacramento Bee*.

In a recent interview in Berkeley, California, Katherine McCamant spoke about cohousing in America—in particular, its appropriateness for midlife and older people.

KATHERINE MCCAMANT

Our search for a new type of life-style has been both a personal and a professional one. As a young married couple living in San Francisco, Charles and I began to think about where and how we would raise our children. How could we best combine our already hectic professional lives with child-rearing? Our relatives lived far away, and our friends were scattered across the city. We dreamed of an affordable neighborhood where we would have friends close by, and our children would have playmates.

When we studied architecture in Denmark several years ago, we were impressed by the Bofaellesskab communities, in which people of all ages lived, and neighbors knew and helped one another. Memories of these small villages kept creeping back into our minds. We knew they made sense, but we realized we would have to learn more about them. Although this type of small community was thriving and successful in the Netherlands, Sweden, France, Norway, Germany, and especially Denmark, nothing had been published about them here.

At that time, I was working for a nonprofit housing developer, encouraging resident involvement/participation in an urban fifty-unit, subsidized family-housing project. We worked on a landscaping project for two years. I soon discovered that this was a good way to build community, even though we had the most diverse group of ethnic backgrounds and languages possible. The success we experienced convinced me that cohousing could work in the United States. .

My husband and I not only thought about ourselves living in such a community, but we thought about Charles's independent sixty-four-year-old mother. She's a widow who raised six kids and continues to work—as she did all of her life. She is a very social person but now feels quite isolated, living alone in the home where she raised her kids. Her neighborhood is not the best—so we are apprehensive about her safety. She's too young for a retirement community, but what are her other alternatives? The family has talked about Charles's sister building a "mother-in-law" apartment in back of her house, but that creates a dependency that neither his mother nor his sister feel comfortable with. Both of us could envision her in a community similar to the one we had seen in Denmark. There she would still be able to work, maintain her autonomy, and be around kids, which she loves. If she wanted to go to a movie, there would always be someone to go with.

People's Changing Needs

We both had designed many types of housing but were amazed at the indifference most housing professionals exhibited to people's changing needs. Developers and banks were used to building for only three segments of the population—single-family detached homes for young nuclear families, condominiums for singles, or retirement villages for older people. Little planning was being done for the quarter of the population who lived alone. We knew more desirable living conditions existed and so decided to spend another year in the Netherlands, Sweden, and Denmark, studying and living in several cohousing communities. Our book, which describes eight very diverse Danish communiites, is the result of this trip.

We returned home to Berkeley to devote ourselves full-time to promoting the idea of cohousing in the United States. We recently began a company to make cohousing a viable option for a lot of people. Cohousing is a term we coined, the mark of our company. It defines a very specific kind of cooperative housing, as described in our book. We have trademarked it because all of a sudden there is a lot of interest in cohousing. It's become this hot, sexy thing, and we're concerned that some developers will begin to toss it around.

We want to make cohousing open to a broader group of people and to make it an easier participatory process. Our new company brings together a team of professionals who first understand development—how to take plans to the bank, how to negotiate the site, and how to get the approval of local planning boards. We also understand the group-participatory process, which most developers won't touch with a ten-foot pole.

The main thing is that cohousing just doesn't happen casually. It's got to be approached in a professional manner. Banks don't want to deal with groups of people. They are scared to death of that. After finding sites, the next hard part is finances. So, what is needed is a financial consultant who knows how to talk bank language, and who is the only one who deals with the bank.

Across this country there are about thirty cohousing groups in process right now, mostly on the West Coast, because that's where we conduct workshops. Others are forming in such places as Rochester, New York, Amherst and Boston, Massachusetts, and in Minneapolis. Cohousing is definitely on its way. We just finished the initial designs for a Davis, California, group, which plans to start construction this summer. A group in Seattle, Washington, is also moving along very fast. Several groups in the San Francisco Bay area are ready to go but are having problems finding affordable sites. We've had letters from up and down the East Coast and from almost every state. In the next two years, I think we'll have several cohousing projects completed and several under construction.

The Cost of Cohousing

You asked me if cohousing is cheaper than bottom-line housing in any given area. We say that cohousing will be in the price range of any cluster housing in any neighborhood you choose. When you look at the cost of housing, it comes down to two factors: the cost of land, materials, and labor and the cost of financing. Sometimes, to bring down the expense, someone will underwrite the cost of the land.

In cohousing, what you do is reduce the size of the individual units and take that space and put it into a large common house. What you get is a viable clustered-housing type for a broad range of people. This is particularly good for families with kids, who would have to choose single-family houses because few condominiums are designed for children. It's also good for people like me who want a garden, which condos don't allow, either. You get a lot more for your money.

Most cohousing groups are urban, even though the land costs are much more expensive, and finding land is very difficult in cities. Groups find a site, can't afford it, and then move on. The way you get a site is to be there day in and day out. If it doesn't work out now, you contact the owner every three months or so to say, "How's it going? We're still interested, just let us know." Maybe in six months, or even two years, they are ready to sell—and they'll come back to you. But it takes someone constantly being on top of things, and it's almost impossible for individual groups to do that. That's one of the services our development company offers.

Cohousing for Midlife and Older People

It has been the goal of cohousing from the very beginning to be intergenerational, which the first projects in Europe were not very successful in doing. I think that's because they began in the early seventies, when there was a lot of suspicion from the older generation about communes, and cohousing was an unknown idea. In those days, when older people came to express an interest in the community, they didn't see any other older faces.

Over the years, cohousing has become a better-known concept, and one of the big draws has been the diversity in age of the people living together. One thing that has helped is the new range in the sizes of units, so that studios and one-bedroom apartments are available. Today, in Denmark, the newer communities have lots more age diversity than the original ones.

On the other hand, everyone in the older communities in Denmark has aged fifteen years. In two of the first rural communities (completed in 1972 and 1973), most of the "children" are now in their early twenties. Several of their parents told us that they were planning to move back into Copenhagen. They still wanted community, but this time in the city, with other middle-age members of their cohousing family. One thing they were clear about was that they had no intention of ever living alone again.

Cohousing for People Over Forty

I think there are tremendous prospects for people over forty in cohousing. In the developing Oakland, California, group, there are several single women in their forties who have never had kids. They don't want to live in a shared housing situation, because they like their autonomy—but their desire for community is equally as strong as their housing needs.

Once, after a presentation, an older woman in the audience raised her hand and said, "We used to have community. Forty years ago when I lived with my husband, if someone moved in, you baked a pie and took it over." My reply to her was that a young couple had moved across the street a year ago, and I'd been thinking about baking a pie—but I don't even have time to bake a pie for myself. That's one of the major changes in how neighborhoods work today. We used to have strong neighborhoods because women were home all the time—and they developed the networks. Now, most women work full-time, and extended families are no longer a reality. That's why supportive networks outside of the family, like cohousing villages, need to be built.

Cohousing for Low-income People

We find that interest in the concept ranges from people who don't know how they'll pay their next month's rent, to people who own half-million-dollar homes. The way you make cohousing affordable is the same way you make any other housing af-

fordable—find local, state, or federal subsidies, get someone to underwrite the cost of the land, or get favorable financing. In East Palo Alto, California, we gave a presentation to a very interested poor black community. We turned the meeting over to them after we showed our slides, and said, "Is this applicable to you—does it make any sense here?" One of the first people to speak up was a young single mother with a six-year-old, who said right away, "What we need is a drug-free community!" We've got poor families all over the country trying to raise kids in deteriorating neighborhoods, when what they need is a strong community. Child care is a huge issue. Women working all day in low-income jobs need some assistance in raising their children. Our aim right now is to get some market-rate cohousing communities built, so that we have good models to demonstrate for funding.

Equity Sharing

I think equity sharing is going to be a good option for cohousing. When someone has a lot of equity in their home and decides to move into a smaller, less expensive cohousing unit, they might have enough money left to help another person struggling to find a down payment. When the house is sold, the equity is split. It's essentially a partnership—one that has been traditionally practiced between parents and children for years.

Rentals

Another idea we have been thinking about is that people in a particular cohousing group, who are moving from larger homes, might want to purchase a second house to rent. Rentals give the community some flexibility. That would have to be set up very carefully, but I'm a believer that if you have good intentions, anything can happen. On any given street in suburbia, there is a spare bedroom used only once or twice a year. In cohousing, we might plan four spare bedrooms for twenty families—and that would be enough. Let's give it a try, and see if it works.

The trick with rentals is how they are financed—initially, who owns them? The best situation we've seen is for a nonprofit organization outside of the cohousing community to own the rentals. Several communities in Europe had short-term rentals. One community had a farmhouse on the property, which they converted to three apartments that could be rented for no longer than two years. For example, one of the men who lived there lost his wife to cancer, and their kids were long gone. He sold his house and moved into the rental apartment at that time to sort out what his next step would be. Sometimes kids come back to live for a while, or a couple may be in the process of divorce and don't want to leave the community. A weekly or day-to-day rental allows for visiting older parents. In one Danish project, *rental guest rooms were owned by the community and called "supplementary rooms." We lived in one when we were doing the research for our book. In another case, a community teenager rented a room for a while. One of the tough things about small housing is living with a teenager. This young man didn't have to leave his home or the community, and the problems were alleviated.*

As pioneers of the American cohousing concept, we have to remember that the first communities are not going to have everything. Every developing group is looking for that perfect mix of people. In Denmark, the first communities were really criticized by the liberals as "ghettos for young families who can afford to own their own homes"—but they were the ones who got the first cohousing built. The next groups added on ideas, as did those that followed. On one hand, I fully support the intergenerational, multi-ethnic group concept. On the other hand, I think that right now in America, we just need to get some projects built. Cohousing offers a new model for re-creating a sense of private space in a caring community.

Getting Started

The process of forming a cohousing community is usually begun by one or two enthusiastic people, who put an advertisement in a local newspaper or post a notice in relevant areas. Interested people meet in workshops to determine their compatibility, decide how they want their project to look, find land on which to build, and then join financial resources. In this "getting started" phase, groups learn about what other groups are doing. They also seek to learn more about one another. Members work on committees of their choice—such as legal, finance, new membership, site selection, housing design, or group activities. The sense of community begins months before construction, as participants join in the design process. Working with experienced architects and designers, the future residents create the layout of their own living space.

Several communities have re-zoned commercial areas and school sites to multifamily residential areas. If those can't be used, some groups renovate an old town-house development. They stress that cohousing is not a synonym for back-to-the-earth communal living. Nor are they like condominium developments, conceived by professional developers and run by an elected board once the units are sold. Condominiums proliferated across this country in the last decade. Too many of them were built, and many are now up for sale. Perhaps in the future some of the smaller condominiums will be adapted to the cohousing concepts.

A core group has at least four basic tasks. The first is choosing a legal structure for the group. Legal structures can range from an informal association to a partnership or corporation.

The second task is developing management capability. Management capability is critical. All lenders will want proof that management is able to complete such a large project—and that financial resources are sufficient to meet the project's needs.

The third task is obtaining construction financing, or the money borrowed to build the project (not the financing of individual units).

Finally, the core group must choose a legal form of community ownership. Ownership of the community should be decided at the very onset. In Denmark, the most common ownership structure is similar to that of a condominium. Individuals have mortgages and own their individual units but share ownership in the common facilities in the form of a residents' association.

An East Coast Architect Gets Started

One person involved with the "getting started" process in cohousing is forty-three-year-old Australian-born architect Bruce Coldham, one of the leaders of the cohousing movement on the East Coast. He is hoping to design cohousing villages in the New England area and to live in one with his wife and four children. They have previously lived in communities in England and Australia before making their home in Amherst, Massachusetts, where I interviewed him.

BRUCE COLDHAM

My office has become an East Coast cohousing company collaborating with Katherine McCamant and Charles Durrett on the West Coast. We are all practicing professionals trying to make a difference by doing something that isn't conventional. I see two roles for myself: one is to promote cohousing so that it sounds intelligent and useful, and the other is to provide services for developing cohousing groups. Each community needs to be differently designed. After groups have chosen a site, getting a good design program should be a high priority.

I think people would be interested in cohousing for four reasons: mutual family support, companionship across the age groups, security (a cohousing community has the best neighborhood-watch system going), and affordability.

People often feel isolated in conventional homes. Cohousing offers community life, conviviality, and a sense of belonging. And it can be accomplished at less cost than conventional housing. I believe in building structures that will allow for expansion as a family grows and changeable use of the space when the children leave home.

What we're really talking about in cohousing is functioning neighborhoods in which you choose your neighbors and they choose you.

Cohousing is also a personal vision for me. Right now I hardly ever speak to my neighbors, let alone cook dinner for them. But in the near future, I see my family building a cohousing community right where we are. We own five acres of land, and the town owns the farmland adjoining it. We would like to get six friends of ours to buy the land, so we could build a small cohousing community clustered around the open field. Our big barn would be a perfect common house.

Financing Cohousing

Cohousing is more affordable because the houses are presold. There are no realtor fees or marketing costs, and future bulk-buying saves money. Building a supportive, caring, and cohesive microcommunity means more disposable income for its constituents, because living costs are lowered.

It's best to go to the banks for private financing instead of becoming involved with all the restrictions of public housing. To the private-banking industry, cohousing is a very salable idea. By the time you approach a financial institution, each family unit in your cohousing group has already made a substantial financial commitment to the process. All the homes you are planning have essentially been presold. It helps to have a member who is experienced in dealing with banks. Most lay people are insecure with banks—not accustomed to saying, "Do I have a deal for you!"

Cohousing for Older People

On their own many older people can no longer handle their yards or painting and repairing their homes. What used to be fun stops being possible. Older people have so much to offer in a cohousing community. I can envision informal swapping, where I might do the heavy work, like shoveling snow for an elderly person, and they might agree to keep an eye on my kids when they come home from school. The two aspects of companionship and security that cohousing offers are especially important for older people. Cohousing works well for people who have just sold their family home and have immediate access to the capital needed.

The Australian granny flat idea [which is addressed in chapter 8] *might work in cohousing. There could be an option to build or import an additional unit for this purpose, whenever a family would need it.*

Possible Problems in Cohousing

Some new cohousing groups will want to do everything for themselves, without hiring a lawyer, developer, or architect. I think this could be a dangerous route, because you don't really know what they would be getting into. Each group should determine what it can do for itself and what professional help it will need. For example, the group might want to hire the California-based CoHousing Development Company to learn about model common-house kitchens. Katherine and Charles have fifty slides of such kitchens—little ones, big ones, fixtures, how to arrange space relationships, and such. This will help groups to become quickly informed and avoid making the mistakes of others.

A second potential problem will be the need to override the zoning regulations of many towns that don't have cluster housing on their books.

People often say, "Me, cook a meal for seventy people? You have to be joking!" I don't see this as a problem. The reality is that in cohousing, they would have to cook only every three weeks, with other people helping. Cooking for many people may seem like an enormous job, but in a spacious, well-equipped kitchen it's much easier. You need only one recipe, because three weeks later everyone is ready for your curry again. And just think of the relief of all the other nights when you can come home and sit down to community dinners filled with interesting discussions.

A problem for the first American cohousing communities (simply because they are pioneers) will be the need to take on the major task of public education. They will be inundated with inquiries from interested people, who want to come visit for a day or more. Each group will have to decide whether it will welcome visitors or not. Too much public attention could interfere with its need to build its own inner sense of community.

Three Cohousing Development Models

In **condominium projects,** the core group forms legal agreements and hires a for-profit developer, a conventional lender provides the money, and ownership comes through individual mortgages.

In **housing cooperative** models, the group acts as a legal entity, which gives them more control over people who buy into the community. The cooperative has a blanket mortgage and makes one monthly payment for the entire community. The financial strength of each individual is no longer critical. He or she owns a share in the corporation, and is thus entitled to occupy a certain unit, rather than owning real property. The value of shares may increase with the years. Transferring ownership becomes less complicated. This model assures a greater degree of participatory management.

In ***models for lower- or mixed-income households,*** the group makes an agreement with a nonprofit developer and obtains financing from public and conventional sources. Residents lease units from the nonprofit developer. The lease could include a clause stating that, in the future, the project might change status from a leasing co-op to a project owned by the group.

Cohousing differs from most of the intentional communities and communes in the United States. These are often organized around strong ideological beliefs and may depend on a charismatic leader to establish the direction of the community and to hold the group together. Cohousing draws much of its inspiration from the increasing popularity of shared households, in which several unrelated people share living quarters. Yet, cohousing is distinctive in that each household has a separate dwelling and chooses how much it will participate in community activities. Again, cohousing will never be like the increasing number of life-care communities for well-to-do older people, which provide on-site health treatment. Cohousing is based on democratic principles and the desire for a more practical and social home environment.

Cohousing, as we have seen, is not without its problems. Although the American founders of cohousing talk about affordability, cohousing seems to be as expensive as other market-rate housing. However, you do get a lot more for your money, with all of the extra space in the common house for child care, workshops, and exercise rooms you could otherwise not afford. Day-to-day living costs are less when you pool resources.

Further, no one knows whether Americans, with their deep-seated desire for individuality and privacy, will accept the premises of cooperation and sharing.

In the last decade, however, our society has learned a lot about group decision making and conflict resolution. Many of the cohousing groups make decisions based on consensus. This method is worth striving for, but sometimes a backup system—like a three-quarters majority vote—is necessary when an immediate decision must be made. Today there are professional mediators who can be brought in to help with difficulties in group decision making.

What Is the Process When Someone Needs to Leave a Cohousing Community?

In cohousing, flexible rules are necessary to allow people to leave easily when they have to. If the project is a condominium model, the house is offered first to people in the community. The seller has an obligation to give notice before selling, which gives the community thirty to ninety days to come up with another buyer. Then, the unit is generally put on the open market, with the community making sure that interested people know that they are buying into a participatory situation.

If the project is a cooperative, the seller does not own his/her house, but a share in the corporation that owns the development. That share goes back to the corporation, and it decides who can buy next. There is very little turnover in cohousing communities, although it is not necessarily a housing type that will suit someone for their entire life. When new people do come in, however, they bring with them a new kind of energy.

• • •

Virginia Barclay Goldstein, seventy-three, is a licensed marriage and family counselor and an art therapist who has been a faculty member of San Francisco State University. She received a BFA from the Chicago Art Institute and a masters degree in counseling from San Francisco State. Virginia is an active member of the Oakland, California, Cohousing Association, and she talked enthusiastically about their progress during a recent interview.

VIRGINIA BARCLAY GOLDSTEIN

I'm seventy-three, and I love to tell everybody. My husband and I live in our own home up in the Oakland hills. My genes are such that I'm going to live to be one hundred—working most of that time, walking and dancing to the end. We have a married daughter living in Sacramento and an eight-year-old granddaughter.

My husband is a professor emeritus at California State in

Hayward, where he taught neurophysiology. His specialty is bioinstrumentation in the medical field. Norman is younger than I am, but he has taken an early retirement because of his health. He's recently been hired to do a writing and research job for the Institute of Noetic Sciences. One of his personal dreams for cohousing is to run a music program, using his enormous collection of audiotapes. He's also a fantastic breadmaker—and would love to teach that to other people. He can't do physical work, but he knows everything about electricity.

All Ages/Diverse Interests

I've always had this idea of community in mind. Even as a young person living in Chicago, it seemed idiotic that those huge apartment buildings were built without some way to prevent every woman from having to cook her own dinner. My dream now is to live with people of all ages, who have a diversity of interests. To be in a community with those who have accomplished whatever it is they were going to accomplish and are doddering on golf greens everyday doesn't appeal to us. We have relatives who talk only about their childhood. Their new ideas are few and far between, and we don't want that for ourselves.

I relate very well to younger people. Most of my friends are in their forties, and they consider me an equal friend, rather than their substitute mother. It's hard when you're older to have friends with young children, but they would be there in cohousing. The playroom in the common house would be close enough for people to keep tabs on their children but far enough away that you could carry on a conversation during dinner.

Norman is not quite as excited about cohousing as I am, but then, I'm the optimist of the family. He's less apt to put time in at this point to make it happen. But he would love to have people coming over casually and frequently, just as his own family once did. We've lost that kind of community—and that might be one of the biggest losses in society today. So really, we are seeking community.

After investigating a few of the cohousing groups in the Bay Area, we've decided to join the one in Oakland. The group got started after a slide presentation about cohousing in Denmark, shown by Katherine McCamant and Charles Durrett. We meet the first Wednesday of every month. The group has about fifty people, some couples, some singles, with a pretty good spread of ages. I think I may be the oldest but by no means the least active.

The Ideal Size for Cohousing

The question is always asked about what size group we would really prefer. In Denmark, one cohousing project that didn't succeed was too small—and problems arise when the group gets too *big. So my ideal would be somewhere between twenty and thirty households.*

We hired someone to come in to teach us how to run meetings effectively, and as a result, our meetings are now smoother and better organized. We also hire one of the teenagers to take care of the children while we are having our business meetings. The whole group pays for that. I am perfectly happy to pay for someone else's child care, to have what I want. We're now working on a values statement and deciding which form of financing is best for us. Then comes design, hard to do when we haven't yet found a site.

In our group, some people will have a studio apartment, and others will need three- or four-bedroom homes. We're beginning to talk about one hundred dollars a square foot, which would include a share of the common space. Norman and I are lucky. We bought our home for $50,000 fifteen years ago, and it's probably worth $425,000 now. The crazy way things are going in San Francisco, a young couple today would have to be earning at least $80,000 to buy their own small home.

Building an Extended Family

The Oakland Cohousing Association has a newsletter that includes a roster of everyone who belongs. If you want to call someone up, it's handy. We also have put together a "family" photo album, with a picture of each member and a personal statement about who they are, what they do, and what they are interested in. It feels so lovely to be able to browse through that and see who our prospective neighbors will be. One is a speech therapist and another is a lawyer. They all have bright and intelligent-looking faces.

We have an occasional party and potluck dinners to get to know one another outside of our working committees. Now when I go to the meetings, I feel as though I really know people. I often quote Charles Durrett when he says: "Take the block I live on. If we all formed cohousing tomorrow, a third of the people I would not be too thrilled with, but I could work with them; a third of them I'd get along just fine with; the other third I'd love to spend time with."

And I think that's probably true. In this situation, it's to your advantage to get along. There's so much known now about conflict resolution and conciliation. If the group is willing to use those methods, we can handle any problems.

Another benefit of cohousing is having people at hand. There have always been people I like, and who I'd like to keep track of, but I do not have time to invite them over for dinner. It's just too hard to plan to get together three weeks ahead of time and then commit four hours to that evening. One thing I look forward to in cohousing is having new friends close by and to be able to invite my old friends for dinner the nights that I'm not cooking—so I can just enjoy them.

We are social beings, and cohousing makes being connected to other human beings easier!

.   .   .

My son John and his new wife, Christina, were given the cohousing book by McCamant and Durrett as an engagement gift. This was the idea they had been looking for. In July 1989, they enthusiastically placed an ad in an Amherst, Massachusetts, paper, which read, "Couple seeks others to buy land and build a community." Twelve people responded. At an initial meeting, they dreamed out loud about the type of community they would like to create. They wanted a rural group of approximately fifteen to twenty households, in which individuals and families could be nurtured and strengthened. They became the Pioneer Valley Cohousing Group.

At each meeting, they have continued to define who they are, what they want from this community, and what obstacles they will have to face to reach their goals. An organizing agreement and bylaws have been completed. The organizing agreement states that people of any sexual preference, religious, racial, or ethnic background will be welcomed. Steps have been taken to ensure intergenerational diversity, by setting four units aside for those over the age of fifty.

A needs-assessment form was completed by members, asking for information about desired site location, style of housing, and specific needs for common space. Each household submitted an annual-income survey. An initial estimate of the costs associated with developing the cohousing project was drawn up. Each household is projected to cost from $85,000 to $127,000 (assuming that there are twenty participating households)—with the cash requirements for each spelled out for year one and year two. Potential financial sources are being explored. Attorneys and architects have been interviewed. A weekend retreat is planned, as well as social get-togethers.

Members have divided themselves into working committees, including membership and outreach, philosophy/decision-making, finance and legal, site design, and the coordinating committee. Committees bring their recommendations to the common meeting, where all final decisions are made.

Prioritizing Needs

In order to prioritize their desires, the group devised the following questionnaire:

Each household has twenty points to award to the features of the common space that are most important to them. You might give one point to a feature you think would be a nice idea, four to a feature you'd like a lot, and fifteen to the feature you wouldn't want to live without. The number of features you choose and the way you disperse your points is up to you, as long as you award no more than twenty points total.

—Kitchen and dining
—Game room
—Art and workshop studios
—Store (staple goods/ food)
—Guest rooms
—Child-care space
—Pillow room (kids' romp space)
—Pool/pond
—Greenhouse
—Garden
—Outdoor barbecue/patio
—Storage
—TV room
—Soundproof music room
—Root cellar
—Laundry
—Performance space
—Sauna
—Hot tub
—Exercise space
—Recycling center
—Children's play area
—Other

The top six choices of participating members were kitchen and dining, art and workshop, laundry, garden, kids' space, and recycling center. The most frequently desired work spaces were workshop, woodshop, garden area, arts/craft space, office space, and child-care space.

The Pioneer Valley Cohousing Group is challenged to "hold in their hands what their hearts could tell." Their process of communicating—challenging assumptions, disagreeing and agreeing, creating solutions, defining, playing—has not been easy, but it has been very exciting. They hope to move into their cohousing community in 1992.

America's First Cohousing Community

Most Danish cohousing communities take between four to seven years from conception to completion. Chris Hanson, a development consultant, and his colleagues in the Winslow Cohousing Group, hope to have their project completed in two and a half years. Located on Bainbridge Island, a thirty-minute ferry ride from Seattle, Washington, theirs will be the first cohousing community to open in the United States.

If all goes according to schedule, twenty-five children and forty-five adults of all ages will move into their traditional Bainbridge farmhouse units in July of 1991. Designed by architect Edward Weinstein, these attached homes will have wood siding and gabled roofs, and will be clustered in three neighborhoods— one with large units and two with one-bedroom apartments. Fourteen months after the first organizing meeting was initiated by forty-four-year-old Chris Hanson, all thirty units were sold.

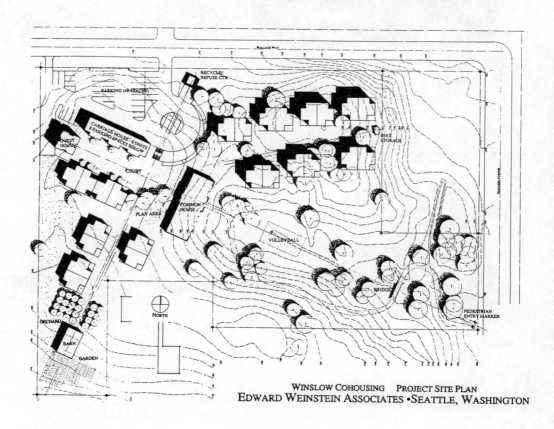

WINSLOW COHOUSING   PROJECT SITE PLAN
EDWARD WEINSTEIN ASSOCIATES •SEATTLE, WASHINGTON

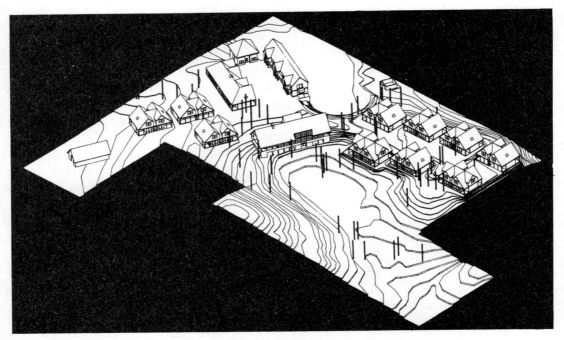

WINSLOW COHOUSING   AERIAL VIEW OF THE SITE
EDWARD WEINSTEIN ASSOCIATES • SEATTLE, WASHINGTON

Aerial view of the site.

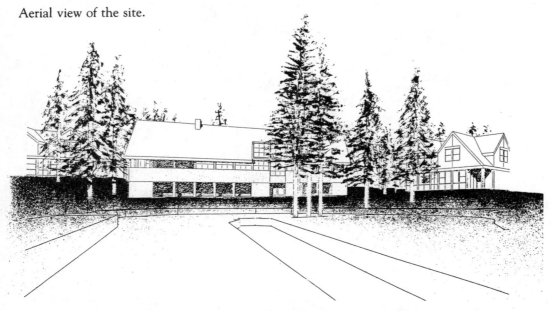

WINSLOW COHOUSING   VIEW ALONG PEDESTRIAN PATH FROM FERRY
EDWARD WEINSTEIN ASSOCIATES • SEATTLE, WASHINGTON

View along pedestrian path from ferry.

Cohousing

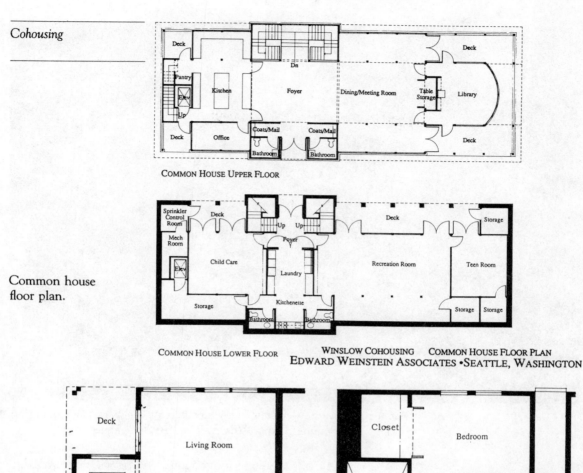

COMMON HOUSE UPPER FLOOR

Common house
floor plan.

COMMON HOUSE LOWER FLOOR   WINSLOW COHOUSING   COMMON HOUSE FLOOR PLAN
EDWARD WEINSTEIN ASSOCIATES •SEATTLE, WASHINGTON

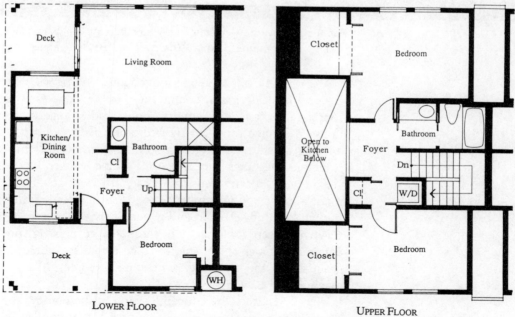

LOWER FLOOR   UPPER FLOOR

WINSLOW COHOUSING   THREE BEDROOM FLOOR PLAN
EDWARD WEINSTEIN ASSOCIATES •SEATTLE, WASHINGTON

Three-bedroom home floor plan.   All illustrations courtesy of Edward Weinstein Associates.

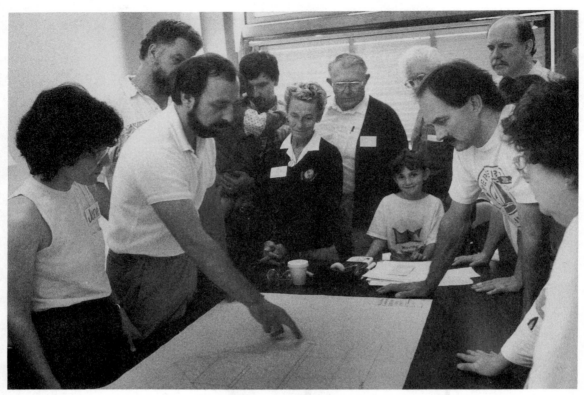

Architect Edward Weinstein with members of the Winslow Cohousing Group. Photographer: Doug Wilson, *The New York Times.*

The 6,000-square-foot common house will contain a dining and meeting room, community kitchen, day-care center, teen room, recreation and laundry room, and storage space. A guest house will have room for six bedrooms. Each adult will pair with another adult to cook once a month. Community dinners will be available five times a week as well as one weekend brunch.

A recent *New York Times* article quotes Paulie Thidigsman, a nurse and a member of the Winslow community (with her husband, an obstetrician and gynecologist) as saying; "At first our seven children thought their parents were moving into a hippie commune. Once they came to some of our meetings and met the group—the majority are professional people, M.D.'s, Ph.D.'s, teachers—they were relieved." [*]

Despite the concept's being in its infancy, thousands of Americans from all over the country have responded enthusiasti-

[*]September 27, 1990, Section C

cally to the possibility of living in a cohousing community. As cohousing is a new concept in the United States, I eagerly await the development of the first completed communities.

It is my belief that this next decade will see cohousing villages spread rapidly around the United States. The time is right for this model, which offers the privacy of one's own home within a self-selected intergenerational community. Whether in cities or in rural districts, our cohousing units will be distinct from their Scandinavian counterparts in ways we cannot yet know. Americans are more diverse than the Danish or Dutch, and our needs and expectations are different. The pioneers of this movement have done us a great service.

Chapter Five

Large Intentional Communities

For this section of the book, my husband and I traveled to Twin Oaks, Virginia, the oldest existing American intentional community; the Sirius Community in Amherst, Massachusetts; and two Emissary communities in Epping, New Hampshire, and Corona, California. We talked to dozens of people, often having meals with community members and staying overnight in one of their guest rooms.

Intentional communities are formed by groups of people who share a commitment to a common purpose and values. Residents usually hold a similar set of philosophical, spiritual, educational, or scientific beliefs that guide their everyday lives. Land, housing, income, and work may be held individually or shared communally. These communities are generally larger than the previously mentioned arrangements of small-group living.

In the book *Builders of the Dawn,* by Corinne McLaughlin and Gordon Davidson, Greg Heuston, of the Stardance Community in San Francisco, says:

> Living intentionally in community requires a considerable commitment to people and a willingness to embrace a *we* consciousness instead of the familiar *I*

consciousness. This does not mean losing personal freedom in deference to group will. In fact, many of the groups I visited were comprised of strong individualists. *We* consciousness means that each person considers what is best for the whole rather than the isolated part. Living successfully in community greatly depends upon willingness to make this shift in consciousness.

Large-scale intentional-community living has existed for centuries. Research reveals that the oldest communities were religious orders. Religious intentional communities, like those of the Amish, the Shakers, and the Hutterian Brethren, have existed in America for most of this century.

The Hutterians, for example, are a Christian pacifist group who trace their roots to the sixteenth century. Thirty-five thousand members, most of them in New York, Connecticut, Pennsylvania, South Dakota, Minnesota, and Manitoba, Canada, live in communities where they work together, pool their resources, and share their lives. They live simply, devoid of the intrusions of television and personal property. Many of the communities are agricultural, although in the 190-acre community in Rifton, New York, 350 members earn their living through the manufacture of children's furniture.

New Age Intentional Communities

New Age intentional communities have a special dedication to personal growth and social change. Many of them are involved in issues of world peace, the energy crisis, nonviolence, reducing consumption, as well as fighting inflation, pollution, and rising health-care costs. Within each community, members are actively working to create sexual and racial equality.

I was surprised to find that, of the intentional communities we visited, only a few had begun to face the issues of aging among their members and in their admission procedures. The core group of some communities seems to have accepted the prevalent myths of aging—to believe that growing older means going downhill physically, mentally, and socially.

The reality is that today's generation of midlife and older

people are healthier, better educated, living longer, and more actively involved with life than any older population in history. They are determined that their extra years of life will be quality years—and for many, that means living in a lively community to which they can bring their considerable skills, talents, and enthusiasms.

Yes, it will be important for intentional communities to ask such questions as, "What would happen if an *older* member became seriously ill with a long-lasting disease, like Alzheimer's? Would we or could we give them the care they needed? What if someone became too frail to carry their share of the workload or financial commitments?" Some communities already had to face these questions. Twin Oaks recently dealt with the long-term illness of a thirty-year-old dying slowly of cancer. The community actively and lovingly supported him until his death.

Many intentional communities are being forced to work out some of their ageist myths, as members reach forty, fifty, and sixty, and as vital older people apply for membership. It was refreshing to read the following statement from Bob Brown of the Clairemont Project in San Diego:

> Several prospective participants in the Clairemont Project are in their seventies, and declare that the spirit of community they are finding in this group is what they've been looking for all their lives. It is obvious to anyone who has given any thought to the issue, that retired persons have a lot to offer community life and have more time and love to contribute than most younger persons. It seems equally apparent that any community will be more stable and healthy the broader its spectrum of ages is.

A Spiritually Based Intentional Community: The Sirius Community (Shutesbury, Massachusetts)

Corinne McLaughlin and Gordon Davidson, the cofounders of the New Age Sirius Community in Shutesbury, Massachusetts, have had twenty-three years of experience living in all sorts of cooperative arrangements. The Sirius Community was inspired by the several years they lived at Findhorn, a large intentional community in Scotland. Corinne and Gordon also visited more than one hundred intentional communities in the United States, and these experiences led them to write the book *Builders of the Dawn*.

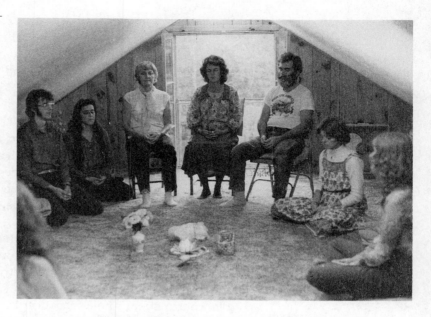

The Sirius Community, Shutesbury, Massachusetts. Above: Sirius Community Meditation. Below: Sacred Dance at Sirius Community. Photographer: Gordon Davidson.

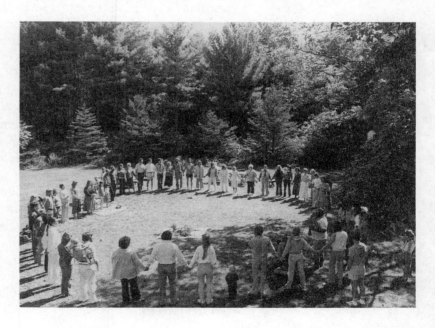

More than a decade ago, they bought eighty-six acres of forest and fields, with a vision "to attain to the highest good in all the levels of God's creation: field and forest, plants and animals, humans and angels, earth and stars." The community calls itself Sirius, after the star known esoterically as the source of love and wisdom for the earth.

The twenty adults and ten children of this rural community have a faith in God, love truth and cooperation, and honor the oneness of life, detachment from desire, meditation, and service to the world. Sirius Community members live in several houses on the land or nearby, and there is a large family of associate members around the country.

Self-governance is by meditative attunement and group consensus, which is described as a sort of spiritual update of the traditional town meeting. Members strive to earn their own living in loving, nonexploitative ways—in such fields as social service, solar construction, whole-foods distribution, land-use planning, and educational services. They grow many of their own vegetables, build their own homes, and heat with wood and solar energy. Full members of the community provide for their own living expenses and contribute equally to the expenses of the land; they share evening meals and maintain a food-buying club.

The Sirius community offers educational programs in community living and spiritual principles, and retreats. Members own several cooperative businesses and organic gardens. They publish *The New England Network of Light Directory* and a *Directory of 440 Communities*.

Individual members take turns planning the weekly Sunday services in any way they feel is appropriate—from contemplative nature walks or sacred dance to devotional singing or discussions of spiritual principles. These services are open to the wider community, and twice a month they are followed by a vegetarian potluck lunch. As a nonprofit educational center, Sirius offers programs on socially responsible investment, solar construction, organic gardening, and spiritual healing, to the public.

Visitors are welcomed from all parts of the world to share a meal, and to join in group meditation and creating solar buildings. Sirius is striving to become a center of light, helping people in their spiritual growth.

I interviewed two members of the Sirius community: Freddie Windriver, a full-time member, and Virginia Senders, an associate member living in the surrounding Hearthstone Village.

FREDDIE WINDRIVER

I'm sixty-one, the mother of three grown children, and recently separated. Like many other women of my generation, I began married life in a nuclear family. Earlier than most people, I discovered community living, starting with an international community in Tokyo. With each transition in my life, I seemed able to find a community to help me build my life. I come from a very small family, and I've longed for a larger family experience.

After five months of living at Sirius, I was sure that it was the right community for me. Since the community is growing faster than spaces can be built (ten people have explored membership in the last six months alone), I temporarily found a house to rent ten miles from the community center. I am the only full member not living within walking distance. But, for now, I am enjoying living alone for the first time in my life and have begun to practice as a private nurse in the area.

When people ask me why I chose the Sirius community, there are many reasons, but the most important one is that its members are consciously building a healing relationship with the earth.

Sirius appealed to me because I was searching for a community that identified itself as spiritual, but one in which political and social-change activism is recognized and celebrated. The acceptance of many spiritual paths among members is an essential component for me. Many points of view are expressed here— Christians, Jews, and Buddhists are free to follow their own paths. Almost everyone believes in reincarnation, astrology, and channeling. Every Sunday we have a meditation for a healing of the planet. My major outside interest right now is with the American Holistic Nurses Association and the Green Movement.''

Welcoming Older People

The Sirius community welcomes older people. One of the exploring members last year was in her sixties; two other people are my age, sixty-one; and several others are in their late fifties. It's not a community of young people. I have worked as a public-health nurse, encountering many older people (usually women) who live alone, and I have ached from the isolation and loneliness they feel. I believe that people who grow old in a caring community will avoid many of the physical and emotional health problems of people who live alone. Here there is an attitude of appreciation and cooperation, which is so important. I think community is a wonderful way to live as you are growing older.

The Membership Process

The process of membership at Sirius begins by getting to know other members—joining them for work days, Sunday services, and meetings. Interested people are invited to attend an orientation group for a few months to decide whether they want to formally explore membership. During this period, they are expected to function as full members. A committee of long-term residents considers one person a month for membership.

Prospective members are told what the committee feels they can best contribute, and what their unique problems and challenges might be. It's a very open, honest balance. They felt my leadership abilities would be important in the community, as well as my experience as a group facilitator and mediator in other community-living experiences. I also have a bachelor of science in nursing. In my private practice I have been able to earn between ten and fifteen thousand dollars a year to pay my own expenses. I contribute fifty dollars a month to the community. All members contribute from their outside income, and a few members are able to earn their income within the community.

Daily Living

Although I live ten miles away, it is a rare day that I don't at least talk to someone from Sirius. I spend Thursday, Saturday, and Sunday there—and some additional time when particular events are going on. Full members are required to attend the weekly business meeting and do eight hours of work for the community each week. We have lots of fun working together on Saturdays. Any guests who are here for the weekend join us. Our major tasks right now are building new housing, planting and harvesting the garden, and doing computer work for our mailing list and publications. Each person chooses what work they want to do.

Recently we formed a choir for healing services, and it feels so nurturing to me to sing with a group of friends. When it's my turn to be responsible for Sunday services, I invite people to share music.

In this community, you eat well and are health conscious. I feel healthier now than ever before in my life. Many members are vegetarian, drink little alcohol, and exercise regularly.

What Next?

Right now I feel that I will be connected to Sirius for the rest of my life. I really want stability and hope that this is the place to find it. My long-term personal goal is to develop some kind of prepaid, holistic health-care system within the community that would be inclusive of all of our needs.

Being a mother and caring about the grandchildren I don't yet have, I feel I must put my energies toward building the beautiful life this planet was created to nourish. I am grateful to Sirius for providing this potential.

An Associate Community

An entire village, called Hearthstone, where more than eighty-five people have made their permanent home, has grown up around Sirius. These associate members of the Sirius Community eat, meditate, and celebrate with full members of the community—and share gardening, parties, and fun.

At Hearthstone, people have the best of both worlds: freedom to travel for long periods of time, independence, and yet the chance to be connected in many ways to the spiritual and educational activities of Sirius. Freddie recommended that I interview Virginia Senders, a Hearthstone resident and an associate member of the Sirius Community. An emeritus professor of psychology at Framingham State College in Massachusetts, Ginny is sixty-five years old, divorced, and the mother of two adult children. The interview took place in her attractive small home.

VIRGINIA SENDERS

In 1972 I spent a thrilling month at Findhorn, in Scotland. The new faces and new things I encountered there were so exciting, and at that time I had what you might call a conversion experience. At any rate, it caused a very radical change in my whole way of looking at psychology, political action, and the world. In the years since, I have been living out those changes.

As soon as I heard about a community similar to Findhorn being founded in Massachusetts, I began to visit it on a yearly basis. It soon felt like my community. I think of it as a New Age think tank. Eventually I became a full member of Sirius and was able to purchase a house just a block away from the center.

For a while I enjoyed the life-style the community offered, including the physical and emotional work that is required there. But I still yearned to live more independently. In 1988 I resigned and moved my membership to the status of associate member and transferred my energies into building an associate community—the Hearthstone Village. We remain closely connected to Sirius. My perception is that Hearthstone Village is the large entity, with Sirius as a small, idealistic entity within it.

A Spiritual Connection

Although we at Hearthstone have chosen to live independently, free from strict community guidelines, the people here continue to put the good of the world and their own personal inner development far ahead of material possessions. They often choose not to take high-paying jobs elsewhere, in order to stay at Hearthstone.

However, the village needs the spirit and energy of Sirius, and if that community were to fade away and die, the village would soon collapse. Some people have moved to Hearthstone Village because Sirius is here. Many are former members who want to remain connected. We share their woodworking shop, the bulk store, dancing space, the sanctuary, and the big garden. We each pay just a dollar a day to have access to any of the fresh garden produce and the foods the bulk store has to offer, like grains, tomatoes, honey, herbs, and more.

One thing that is very important to me is the daily community dinner, joining members of Hearthstone Village and Sirius. At the beginning of each month, you sign up for the nights you want to participate. It's a movable feast, with dinner moving from house to house. Last night it was my turn to cook, and fifteen people came to dinner. When it is your turn to cook you also pay, shop, and clean. Another way the people in the village remain connected to each other is through the biweekly newsletter The Hearthstone Cricket, which I organized and edit.

Three of the houses in the village are group homes. We formed a community land trust to buy one house when it went on the market; it now has six young singles living in it. We have a community copy center, a Macintosh computer, and a laser printer.

At Hearthstone, everyone follows some kind of spiritual discipline. We celebrate equinoxes, solstices, and full moons. We rejoice with one another and offer support in times of need. We trust one another and rejoice in our interdependence. We spawn enterprises—a land trust, a community office, a health-food business, a massage practice, a catering service, cooking instruction, an insulation business, and a recycling program. We are concerned with local government, as well as with global justice and planetary healing.

What Next?

I am one of those people with a strong superego. I have been exceptionally fortunate and therefore feel that I have exceptional *responsibilities. I just returned from a second "peace" trip to Nicaragua and a trip to the Soviet Union with Interhelp. I'm on the board of directors of Temenos, a local retreat center, and on the board of Wainwright House, a New Age center. I also do some private therapy. It's a real privilege to be a companion on someone's journey, someone you can honor with intense listening and attention and the willingness to hold back on answers so that they can work their own way through.*

I have almost too much going on in my life right now, leaving me little time to paint, hike, or mountain climb. In my entire life there were maybe two years when I wasn't working, so I'd like to plan more time for these hobbies in the years ahead. I feel retirement should be the time you say yes to all the things you had to say no to all of your life.

People my age move to a retirement village because they don't want to live alone. Unfortunately this means living with only one age group. At Hearthstone, I neither live alone or with people of one age group. I am the oldest person living in the village by fourteen years. I would be thrilled if your new book resulted in a few older people moving to Sirius. I would like to have some over-sixty companions, male and female. Right now, housing is the problem. But I can imagine an apartment with, say, six private dwellings, that would attract older people.

What I would like to say to the people who you are writing for is, there are lots of very enriching ways you can live. You don't have to live in a big old house alone and be lonely. You can and will grow continually in this type of community.

(Interested readers can contact the Sirius Community, Baker Road, Shutesbury, Massachusetts 01072; 413-259-1251. *Builders of the Dawn*, a book on New Age communities by Corinne McLaughlin and Gordon Davidson, is available from the Sirius Community.)

An Economically Based Intentional Community: Twin Oaks

Twin Oaks, in rural Virginia, is one of the oldest surviving communities in the United States. It was established in 1967 as a model social system, inspired by B. F. Skinner's novel, *Walden Two*. All income, land, homes, businesses, and most resources are shared.

There are six large residences, a children's building, three industrial buildings, and a new large community center/dining facility, built on four hundred acres of land in Louisa, Virginia. All buildings are solar designed and are energy efficient.

At present Twin Oaks is a community of seventy adults and twelve children, with members ranging in age from newborn to fifty-seven years. They are a very diverse group. Twin Oaks is economically self-sufficient and considers itself to be a modern alternative to a "competitive and consumption-oriented society."

The community supports itself by sharing all income and labor from several cottage industries and services, including hammock- and rope-furniture making, indexing for publishers, rope manufacturing, and farming. From 60 to 70 percent of all food consumed (vegetables, dairy products, meat, fruit, and some grains) is produced there. Members provide such services for the community as auto maintenance, sewage treatment, and construction.

All work is divided equally among the members, in a nonsexist way, and everyone does work of their own choosing as far as is reasonably possible. Each member works an average of forty to fifty hours a week in a humane work environment. Within the set of jobs and skills necessary to run Twin Oaks, no member need choose a single skill to make a living; many split their work into several different tasks. Laundry and child care are "paid" the same as vehicle repair or computer programming. At first, forty hours may seem like a long work week; however there is no time spent commuting, and although each person does one specific job, all other typical family needs are taken care of by community members. Integration of work and play is an important goal. The nearby South Anna River provides swimming, fishing, and boating. Members enjoy a darkroom, pottery studio, and woodshop and often take vacations together. The community celebrates the changes of season, and this year, their twentieth anniversary was the occasion of week-long festivities.

Twin Oaks members also have a good relationship with people in nearby towns. They share their skills and talents, offer lectures on community living, and make their publications available. Some members have become involved in local, national, and international political activities.

New Membership

Membership is open, and the community is looking for new people with whom they can share their dreams and goals. Afternoon tours for people who are interested in investigating this life-style are scheduled on Saturdays. Before being accepted for full membership, prospective members must visit for three weeks and then live at

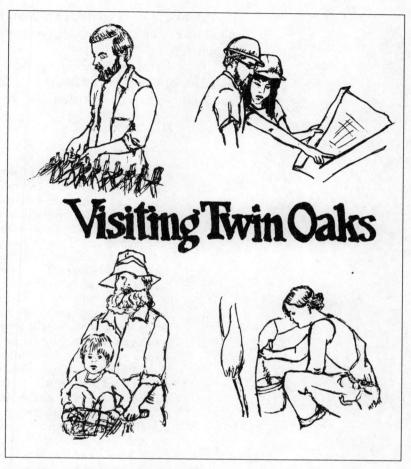

Twin Oaks Community, Louisa, Virginia.

Twin Oaks for a six-month provisional period. Members are guaranteed an equal share of all the benefits the community can provide, in an environment that is neither violent, racist, sexist, nor competitive.

To maintain a sense of equality, new members are expected to share everything except furnishings for their own rooms and other personal possessions. They can keep resources outside the community but are not allowed to use them while living at

Twin Oaks. It costs no money to join. Food, rent, a small monthly allowance, and other basic necessities are provided by the community.

Kathleen Kinkade, age fifty-six, is one of the founding members of the Twin Oaks Community. I interviewed her in the community's large, sunny dining room.

KATHLEEN KINKADE

At the time I read Walden Two, I was thirty-four years old, divorced, raising a child, and making a living working at an office job that I was bored with and found meaningless. I was slowly working toward my B.A. degree at night school, when I discovered the novel in a philosophy course. For me it was a brilliant flash of light! I cannot exaggerate the excitement I felt as I read it. The community it depicted was everything I had ever wanted. It was impossible to believe that it was only a novel, that there was no such place in real life.

I had been searching for an environment where I could find more interesting people to talk to, people with similar intellectual backgrounds. Whatever else brings people to community, the hope of a compatible mate or a close, warm group of friends is usually just underneath the surface. The most sought after dream is the dream of no longer being lonely.

It was not in my plan to be the founder of a community, I just wanted to join an existing one! But Walden Two was a model I was determined to work for. I searched for a few other interested people, and finally someone put up the money to buy the land. Two years later, with seven associates, I began to live on the land. I was the oldest of the group, and my thirteen-year-old daughter was the youngest.

My marriage did not survive this social experiment. The poverty stage at the beginning and the lack of autonomy were difficult for many people, including my second husband. I loved what I was doing—solving questions about how to organize a labor credit system and learning how to ensure equality. My daughter always shared my enthusiasm for Twin Oaks and left only recently to begin her medical internship.

Although I am the only remaining original member of the community, I too left Twin Oaks for five years to build a similar community and to explore other options. For four years I did all the things I hadn't been able to do. And yet, I found myself thinking about Twin Oaks often. When members came to visit me and talked about the process of the community, I would feel alive and excited. I decided to come back.

The variability of the work scene and the fact that I work where I live are two of the major advantages to my life at Twin Oaks. The last time I had a job in the outside world, I was a computer programmer. It was my responsibility to stay in an office for eight hours a day, to sit in one spot and communicate with a computer. This was intellectually challenging, but I found that my knees started to ache, and then my shoulders. My concentration was affected, and yet I was only fifty. Now, doing the same computer programming here at Twin Oaks at age fifty-six, if my knees begin to hurt I can lie down and take a long nap, go to lunch, or do several other things before returning to the office. I can work in the afternoon, the evening, the middle of the night, early in the morning, or on Sunday. All I have to do is put in a certain number of hours each week.

I have many roles at Twin Oaks—manager, clerical person, articulator, and politician/stateswoman. Politics is the art of the possible. I sense what is possible and try to implement that for the good of the community. My own special community here is the leadership group—the people who are interested in bettering Twin Oaks, who continue to think of where and how we need to grow. Unlike some leaders of movements, I'm not charismatic— and feel the community is better off without me, or anyone, trying to act as a charismatic leader. A lot of faith in human nature is necessary at Twin Oaks. We can't solve all problems but we can, given time, make things better, and that keeps us excited.

Twin Oaks and Older People

You asked me how I feel about Twin Oaks as a home for people in the second half of life. We have recently been receiving applications from an increasing number of people over forty. The advantages are clear. When they find they fit in, they say, "Hey, this is nice. There's a lot here for me."

Early on there were so few of us, and we hadn't the faintest idea that we would grow old—age wasn't part of our planning. Even though the average length of stay is four years and the average age is thirty-four, we have twelve members over the age of forty, and nearly a dozen more who will reach their fortieth birthday in the next few years.

Twin Oaks takes care of all the things we are no longer able to do if our bodies weaken. I don't have to do anything I don't feel capable of doing physically. We have a system of pension credits; for every year we are over fifty, we have to do one hour less of work each week. Our oldest member, sixty-three, works only thirty-four hours a week, compared to the forty-seven-hour norm for everyone else. She and I are the oldest members, and we feel we are trailblazers; the community trusts our aging experience.

If I had some disability that meant I couldn't work, I would simply not work, and I'd still be fully entitled to community support. I'm taken care of—that's guaranteed; our social security is absolute. It starts at birth and ends at death and takes care of absolutely everything in between. Even if I had Alzheimer's disease, the community would take care of me. I don't have a doubt in the world about that.

Among the things that concern me now is the heavy selection process at Twin Oaks. I want to accept as many people who might fit in, as many people as we can possibly manage. This isn't a country club! We would like, ideally, in the next decade to have two hundred members (originally our plan was for a thousand).

We also have to change our ideas about family life. We've learned the hard way that families need more living space, and children need their own school.

Twin Oaks is designed for a very narrow segment of the population. It can be difficult to live by community rules and to seek community approval for things from vacation time to personal purchases. It wouldn't work for people who put a lot of emphasis on material goods. We are a sharing community.

At times I feel isolated from younger members. This has to do with different interests spanning from intellectual discussions to their tastes in music and food.

What Next?

My other dreams for the community are cultural. I'd like to see a little orchestra and a real choral group. We have some very talented members. Once a year we have an art show and are surprised at how great the art is. We give work credit here for anyone teaching other members—and art is a part of that.

I recently proposed that we construct our next building with those of us who are aging in mind—all on one floor, no lofts, no stairs, no kids, automatic heating, and a laundry. I'm going to want these as I get old.

If you are a person over forty who wants to look into living communally, you would probably find that Twin Oaks has a lot to offer. I call this a commune that works. I think many of us are here to stay for life.

Kathleen Kinkade speaks about the beginnings of Twin Oaks and about the community's leadership. Joanna Reese brings a more personal view about day-to-day life in this intentional community. Joanna, fifty-seven, was our hostess. We slept in her room, ate three meals together in the dining room, and were taken around the community under her cheerful guidance. Joanna has lived at Twin Oaks for only three years. She says: "All of my roots have led me here."

JOANNA REESE

I lived in a traditional marriage for twenty-three years. I was a housewife in a suburban community, and when my marriage ended, I was left with no career skills, $30,000, and minimal child support.

The years that followed were difficult ones. I suffered the loss of my fifteen-year-old son and was struggling financially as well. My older son urged me to return to college with him. At forty-six, I was admitted to Friends World College, where I completed my degree in a year.

Even with my college degree, I was only able to earn about $10,000 a year. I tried hard to make it out in the world, but like many women, I was in very bad economic straits. I was afraid of becoming like all the hundreds of women around me who lived their own little lives in their own little spaces—went out to a job and came home at night to a cat and a garden. I felt that my life had to move in a new direction.

The beginnings of my living in community came when I moved into an activist life center at the Movement for a New Society (MNS), in Philadelphia, where I lived for two years. This was a priceless, growing time. I lived in an intergenerational house, and twelve of us formed a support group called WOW (Wonderful Older Women).

I began to read everything I could find about larger communities all over the world, including Twin Oaks. I believe that when you are ready to take advantage of something, the "wind just blows you along." I spent three weeks at Twin Oaks as a visitor and immediately applied for provisional membership. Here was a group trying to live differently from the outside world, with a minimal use of material things, and lots of camaraderie.

Day-to-Day Life

I have my own room at Twin Oaks, as does each other adult. We've designated the first floor of my house as women's space. I like living in the midst of women. I eat dinner with others in our new, large dining room but usually have breakfast and lunch in my own room.

What I like best is choosing what I want to do each day. I can set my own pace; very little work is assigned. Because I am fifty-seven, I am expected to work forty hours a week, seven less than the average worker. I'm co-manager for my house, assigning work details and seeing that the house provisions are bought. I am also manager for our indexing business and a member of the health team.

People can work on one project as long as they enjoy it, and then they can switch off. I've learned a step of hammock making, tried my hand at vehicle repair, and recently learned how to repair small appliances, like toasters and irons. Above all, I want to continue to be an involved, productive member of the community.

Every week there is an informal community get-together, a video night, and a dancing evening. The younger people seem very welcoming of my companionship. Several of us have been quilting together, and a neighbor leads a weekly choir. I recently took a vacation with nine other members. We don't gather often enough just for fun as a community, and I feel we need to join adults and children more often.

Each of us has our own personal support groups within the community. We have formed a "wisecracker" group of people over forty and a women's group that supports me and allows me to support others. Women here encourage the feminist side of men, and a men's support group has just been formed. We also tenderly care for members in illness and throughout their lives. I've done a lot of learning in these three years at Twin Oaks.

Problems

One of the problems I find at Twin Oaks is that there is too much work and not enough fun. Even though I know this is a self-supporting community, I believe we all need some chunks of time for creative work, music, and art—and some support from the community for such activities. I also feel the need for more of a spiritual community at Twin Oaks.

I am concerned about the small number of minority people and older people at Twin Oaks. I feel we need a greater race and age span. Having vital older women and men coming to live here would be great.

I often think about what I would do if my eighty-year-old Mom became disabled. Could I persuade her to live here? Would the community object to having her here? These are all things to be worked out in the future.

What is hard is when people leave. About 20 percent of our members leave each year, and almost that many new people join. Constantly forming new friendships is difficult.

Wider Community Links

There is some social activism here, which is important to me. A "Movement Support Group" meets once a month. We support a women's rape center in Charlottesville, joined the local commu-

nity in a fight against having nuclear waste travel through our community, and we bring five gallons of our milk each week into Louisa's senior center. We have agreed to have a young family from San Salvador live with us, setting up bond money for them, and acting as their support group.

A Message to Older People

My message for other women and men in their middle and later years is to know that there's plenty of good life ahead. You have to be strong, have faith, and dare to risk trying new things.

Twin Oaks is a founding member of the Federation of Egalitarian Communities, a group of intentional communities with similar goals and values.

(Interested readers can contact Twin Oaks Community, Louisa, Virginia 23093; 703-894-5126.)

Other *Walden Two* communities have been founded in Kansas, Michigan, Canada, and northern Mexico. The last is the smaller sixteen-year-old "Comunidad los Horcones," an isolated ranch in the desert of northern Mexico. It is home to twenty-nine adults and eleven children, who regard themselves as scientists involved in a long-term research project. It is their belief that human beings can be taught to "build a society based on cooperation and not competition, on equality and not discrimination, on sharing and not individual property, on pacifism and not aggression."

Philosophically Based Intentional Communities: The Emissary Communities

My husband and I visited two Emissary communities at opposite corners of the United States—Green Pastures Estate in New Hampshire and Glen Ivy in California. Although we had never before heard of the Emissaries, we soon discovered that they have built communities on four continents, with some three thousand members; five in the United States, three in Canada, and one each in South Africa, Australia, England, and France. Although each community, with eighty to four hundred people, is as unique as the culture it thrives within, all share a common purpose and direction. People come to Emissary communities after reading their books, attending public meetings held by Emissaries in different cities, and observing television and magazine interviews. Many people also come because of personal contacts.

The Emissaries were founded in 1930 by Lloyd Arthur Meeker. The term "emissary of divine light" refers to those with a stable, true, and loving spirit who bring light to others. It was difficult for me to pin down the Emissary philosophy. All of the Emissaries I spoke to told me that their way of life was neither a creed, dogma, nor a set of beliefs! However, they are recognized as one of the largest and wealthiest twentieth-century religious movements. Around the world, Emissary chapel services are held four times a week (Green Pastures is registered as a church in the State of New Hampshire).

Michael Exeter, who is the international coordinator and spokesman for the Emissaries, lives with his wife at 100 Mile House, in British Columbia. With input from executive and regional councils located around the world, he makes decisions and provides spiritual counsel for all Emissary communities. Respected elders, many of whom are living at 100 Mile House, are also consulted. When I asked about the hierarchical structure, members said that it is much like a family.

"Harmony" is an important word in the Emissary philosophy—harmony in their individual and collective lives, and in the world—and I heard it frequently. The goal of each community is to provide a setting for people to experience their creative potential and to discover the experience of friendship and an ease in living.

Emissary communities hold seminars, classes, and conferences for members and visitors from all over the world. These include one-day art-of-living seminars, weekend study groups, and one- to three-week classes to develop skills in spiritual leadership. Seven communities, including Green Pastures, run Stewardship Farms, a network of farms dedicated to the stewardship and regeneration of the land. The two communities I visited were quite different, both in appearance and in life-style patterns.

Green Pastures Estate

Green Pastures Estate, in southern New Hampshire, was established as an Emissary regional center in 1963. It is located on 160 rural

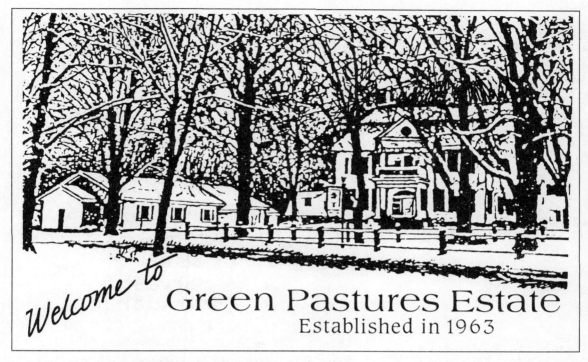

Welcome to **Green Pastures Estate**
Established in 1963

Green Pastures Estate, Epping, New Hampshire.

acres of beautiful woodland, streams, orchards, farms, and gardens, just one hour from Boston. As we drove in, it looked like a small New England village. Considered an educational site, Green Pastures attracts people from all over the world to its seminars and spiritual leadership classes.

Eighty-five people live here, ranging in age from eight to eighty-four. About a third work professionally in the surrounding cities, whereas the remainder work at tasks within the community, including a small forklift repair business. Members, with their diverse talents and experiences, come from different parts of the country. They live in six large and very beautiful white colonial homes. They believe that each person is responsible for managing his/her own life, with proper regard for the rights of others—not just to get, but to give.

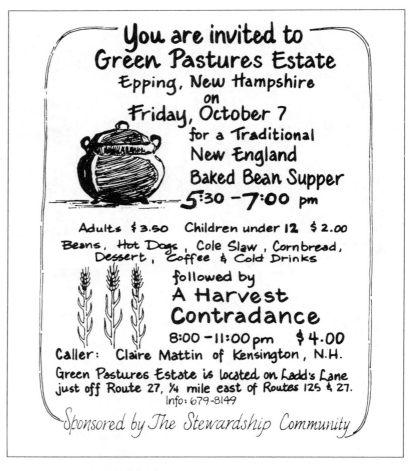

Invitation to a New England Supper.

My husband and I were enormously impressed by the friendliness and openness we found at Green Pastures, from the first person who gave us directions to those we met as we toured the homes and farm. We ate three meals in the communal dining room, and each time several people came over to greet us. They seemed to be unrushed and to enjoy their work (for example, the cooks and clean-up crew were singing in the kitchen). A large and very beautiful chapel is under construction. Every part of the community, both inside and out, was spotlessly clean and well kept, with homes surrounded by lawns, trees, and gardens. A good-sized pond has been dug for summer swimming.

Members are very connected to the local community and have a beautiful exchange with the townspeople. Their children are educated in the local public schools. Emissaries hold positions on the town and school boards and are volunteers for the local fire department. Every year they invite neighbors and friends to two nights of Christmas concerts. Last year, more than four hundred people attended.

David and Diane Pasikov are the coordinating couple of Green Pastures, responsible for the people who live there and all the varied activities. They are in their early forties and have a young son.

When I interviewed David, he explained that the community was supported through a minimal "rent" paid by the members working on the outside, by fees from workshops and seminars, and through donations. He felt that the major challenges he faced in the community revolved around interpersonal relationships and issues of privacy for individual members, particularly in the summer, when many visitors come to workshops.

One of David's main responsibilities is spiritual leadership. He reads Michael Exeter's printed or videotaped sermon each Sunday (the same one that is read and discussed in *every* Emissary community). This week, Michael's message was on being nonjudgmental, and the community tried to put it into practice as they interacted during the week.

Sixty-year-old Alice Penfield moved into Green Pastures some twenty years ago, as a recently separated wife and mother of four. I interviewed Alice in one of the colonial homes that contained six other living units. She has a sunny kitchen, which spills into a dining/living area, and a patio. Her apartment has two bedrooms and contains most of her own furniture, plants, and paintings. She says: "When I tapped into the Emissary ministry, my youngest was two. I lived in a nearby town and came several times a week for a few years to services, classes, and social events. Long before I lived here, Green Pastures felt like my home."

Alice has had the unique good fortune of having her brother and his family live at Green Pastures. And both of her parents lived out their final years in this community. The Emissaries graciously joined with Alice and her brother to support her parents until their death.

ONE WOMAN'S VOICE: ALICE PENFIELD

On a typical day, I have my breakfast at home and go off to do community work in the office for about four hours. After lunch with my friends, I return home to work on a history of Green Pastures, which I have been writing for several months. The living here is healthy, with lots of care given to cooking nutritious and delicious meals and to exercise (I walk or ride my bike every day).

Services are held four times a week. People from the nearby communities often join us, and after services we have lunch, and everyone works together in the garden or on the latest building project. I have built many close relationships in the years I've lived here.

The way I see the Emissary communities is that they have given humankind a nucleus of people who are willing to work at living together. In some sense, we're building a new society. People are open-hearted here. I feel a sense of fullness in myself. I feel like a complete person.

Perhaps my favorite part of visiting Green Pastures was the informal group interview with women over forty. We talked while snacking on popcorn, apples, wine, and soda and were delighted to be together. They spoke with great candor about why they had chosen this community.

If there's one thing that comes from the letters that pour in, it's that people have a hard time making connections—and it's lonely out there for many of them. I grew up in a community with a close-knit group of people who dropped in on each other and frequently had potluck dinners in their backyards. Today, in apartments and condos, people don't even know the names of their next-door neighbors. At Green Pastures we do know our neighbors; we feel like a family and accept one another exactly as we are. That's the part I love best—people close to home who really care about each other. We make very tender-hearted connections here.

◆　◆　◆

I never thought I would live in a community with eighty-five people and love it. I couldn't envision it—it wasn't in my life plan. It all began in my new chiropractic practice, when I wanted to allow patients to set their own fees. Everyone thought I was just a young idealist. Then I met a man who had been doing this for twenty-five years, and he happened to be connected with the Emissaries. So, here I am, seven years later. My parents are very orthodox Jews, but they love to spend time here, and do so often. Even if I'm working, they have a grand old time. They love the spirit of this place.

◆   ◆   ◆

Two years ago I contracted breast cancer—and that made me take stock of my life. I realized that having a spiritual way of life was important to me. The Catholic church I'd grown up in didn't offer any sense of community. So I began to come to services here and to lots of events and classes, and I loved the friendliness of the people and the beauty of the surroundings. Soon I realized that this was where I wanted to live.

◆   ◆   ◆

I would be quite happy living out my life at Green Pastures, but, honestly, I don't think that far into the future. I try to live fully in the moment and not drag my past along with me. Every older person living here is contributing to the community. There's an appreciation of growing older, that older people have not only experience, but a much deeper quality to share. We need older people as much as we need teenagers! We don't send them out to nursing homes and hospitals! They are supported in a lovely way as they complete their life cycles.

◆   ◆   ◆

We didn't choose one another to live with. We just all found ourselves here, because we had a common purpose in life. Then the friendships naturally developed. Part of the attraction for me is that people are not into a "getting" mode, but a "giving" mode.

(Interested readers can contact the Green Pastures Estate, Ladd's Lane, Epping, New Hampshire 03042; 603-679-8149.)

Glen Ivy Emissary Community

News about my book was spreading through the community network, and soon I had a letter from a middle-aged woman who was interested in options for older women in intentional communities. She asked to meet with me.

We met at my apartment in New York City, where she told me about her personal search for community. Sara is a divorced woman in her early fifties and has a masters degree in marriage and family counseling. She had been attending conferences on living in community and wrote her master's thesis about interpersonal and ideological problems in intentional communities. It seemed as if finding the right community had become her life's work.

I met Sara again two years later, at the Glen Ivy Emissary Community in Corona, California, where she has been living for six months. She shares a room and works in what she calls "the house pattern," doing gardening, landscaping, and kitchen and nursery work. She says:

> *California is my home. I resonate in this environment. All my life I've been looking for what I've found here. I kept thinking that it could exist, but I didn't know if it did. When I was five, I remember dreaming about a place with palm trees, red-tile roofs, and octagonal houses—and here they are! I've visited many communities throughout the country and always found one thing lacking—and that was integrity. People were not "walking their talk!" Here I don't have to feel as though I'm walking on eggshells; disagreements are immediately dealt with.*

Unlike Green Pastures, Glen Ivy is a sophisticated business community. Located one hour from Los Angeles, it is home to seventy-five Emissaries of all ages, and it is the coordinating center for Emissary activities in the western United States, Latin America, and the Pacific Rim.

A warm climate and an abundant water supply allow for year-round production of fruits and vegetables. Palm trees, flowers, and bougainvillea surround the homes, which are typical of the colorful villas of the area. The community owns two main residential buildings; one contains the main lodge, a communal dining room, a kitchen, laundry facilities, and two resident floors. Some members have built their own small homes, which the community will inherit. The second building is a residence for members. All but one of the members live and work at Glen Ivy.

Glen Ivy is well known for its hot springs resort and spa—a business owned and run by the Emissary community. Here, wealthy people come to be pampered for the day, using the warm thirteen-mineral pool baths, a red-clay mud bath, sauna, massage, facial treatments, pool swimming, sunbathing, and a snack-bar lunch. People visit Glen Ivy from all over the world. The week I visited, guests were arriving from South Korea, South Africa, Israel, and the Soviet Union.

There is an "adjunct" group of Emissaries in San Diego who live in separate homes and have professional jobs but meet together once a week. This group frequently attends events at Glen Ivy.

The coordinators at Glen Ivy are John and Pam Gray, a couple in their early forties. Their role in the international Emissary community is similar to David and Diane Pasikov's. I had tea with Pam in their lovely apartment. She spoke about how her elderly parents had been cared for by the community; they were able to die at home, close to their loved ones. No older person here is sent to a hospital or nursing home to be cared for by a stranger with no concept of the spirit of life.

A Married Couple at Glen Ivy

One forty-plus couple, Kathryn and Terry, spoke to me about married life at Glen Ivy. They had always been concerned about how to help the world change, and for many years thought that could be accomplished in the corporate world. However, they began to feel that their skills and influence would be more valuable on the grass-roots level, so Terry retired from the computer industry at age forty-one, and they joined the Glen Ivy community.

Now they feel that they are making a difference in the world as they learn to live in community. Here, they do the kind of work they feel is so important, teaching seminars and classes. They receive a modest salary, but all overhead expenses, like food, lodging, and utilities, are taken care of. Because they work and live at Glen Ivy, retirement hasn't had to mean lowering their standard of living.

I asked Kathryn and Terry how living as a couple in community was different. Kathryn responded:

> *To live in community, people have to have created stability in their own lives. They need to have a clear perspective of their own identities and purposes. The time we spend together now, as a family, is different. Dinner used to be one of our main family times, but here the whole community gathers then, so we can't really rely on that as an opportunity to be together. We never have to ask the question, "What will we do tonight?" We thought that when we moved into this community, we would be spending lots of time together. But what we find is a larger variety of options, people, and activities available to us. We see more of each other, but we are not alone much. One danger is that you might avoid doing some of the nurturing things needed in a good married relationship. Now more than before, we have to be conscious of the quality of the time we spend together.*
>
> *About twelve couples live at Glen Ivy. We support one another in a couples group. Women, men, and kids have their own support groups.*

As at Green Pastures, a group of women over forty gathered to meet with me at Glen Ivy. They were bright and articulate—I could have listened to their stories for hours. Perhaps the woman who impressed me the most was a forty-year-old who had just moved to Glen Ivy.

> *I have two reasons for being here: first, to provide an example of creative living for people throughout the world, and second, because the Emissary community supports people in the work they really want to do. I act as a liaison between the American and Soviet film communities. I do a lot of work in different parts of the world and believe that people need to see a life-style based on spiritual values that really works. The Soviet Union is very interested in the Emissary way of life. They have a history of communal experiences that have not been so great. For them to look to the West for an experience of community that is viable, happy, and voluntary is quite a revolutionary thing.*

The oldest of the women I met with was seventy-five and lives with her husband in a small house they built on Emissary land. She said, "We've been here for nine years, and life gets more beautiful every year. I've just gone through radiation treatments and feel totally supported by the community. I believe that the secret for growing older gracefully is to be in love, to give love and to share love."

Many of the women were single and came to Glen Ivy to find family.

> *I never felt that I fit in anywhere, so all through my formative years I was searching. When a friend of mine began raving about this place, I came to explore. It seems clear to me that this is where I belong. I was looking for home and family. Here, I cook, do lots of laundry, garden, and have begun the process of becoming a watercolor painter. But more important than what I do is being with friends. It gives my life fullness to be among people who want the same things—people who want to express their best in their daily living.*

A divorced forty-four-year-old woman loves the range of responsibilities she has been able to assume in her nine years at Glen Ivy:

> *From a professional viewpoint I find here the possibility of exploring almost every avenue of interest and to be with people interested in a larger context of living. Quite early on in life, I discovered that there had to be something more to being on earth than so many of the people I was involved with believed.*

I asked these women what problems they encountered at Glen Ivy. Their answers were very candid:

> *Everything that comes up in the outside world comes up here. We're not exempt from tensions—but the context for them is different. We all have an understanding that this is a microcosm of the world. We have cultural conflicts all the time, but we know that if these things are handled with care, we will find a workable*

solution—a new way to function. We have classes in interpersonal communication and welcome the opportunities for conflict resolution, knowing that our problems aren't just personal but represent something bigger. What we're doing is, in a sense, a world service.

◆　◆　◆

Coming into a community like this, you find that a lot of your personal preferences have to go by the wayside. The way you want things, the way you've always had things, doesn't always fit. We run up against that over and over again. But I see this as growth, giving us a new ability to work with any people, anywhere. There needs to be a lot of give and take, giving other people the space they need. Sometimes we go through painful emotional cycles, but when they are worked out, I feel so good about myself.

◆　◆　◆

Nobody is here because it's comfortable or a better life-style. We're here because there is a spiritual contribution that we can make to the world through our lives together.

◆　◆　◆

Every community is a laboratory for something. And this is a laboratory for spiritual identity and creation. Although we have these magnificent people in this magnificent setting, there would be no reason to be here if we weren't going deeper to discover the meaning of spirituality and embody it in our lives. My own spiritual capabilities change as I grow older. Physical things have become less important, and I have found a new, maturing sensitivity to the things happening in the world around me. Here our usefulness increases as we age.

(Interested readers can contact Glen Ivy, 25000 Glen Ivy Road, Corona, California 91719; 714-735-8701.)

Although Green Pastures and Glen Ivy are different in many ways, the forty or so people I spoke to in both communities were very much alike. All of them lived in community because they chose to, and all of them have the freedom to leave whenever they want.

• • •

One of the secrets of the successful intentional communities seems to be contained in the old saying, "Birds of a feather flock together." And perhaps that is the challenge of all people seeking creative community—to find a functioning group of like-minded people, draw them together, and with them build a new community.

Chapter Six

Traditional Housing Options

FIRST WOMAN: "I'm planning to have a hippy-dippy retirement
community for me and my unmarried friends. Want to join?"
SECOND WOMAN: "Sounds good, but someone has already in-
vited me to join hers. She says it will be veggie-weggie."
FIRST WOMAN: "I'll make mine hippy-dippy *and* veggie-weggie."
SECOND WOMAN: "You're on!"
—*New York Times* "Metropolitan Diary," February 2, 1990

Maturing people looking for traditional housing options fall into four subgroups: people over forty moving to warmer climates; older single people and couples looking for smaller, maintenance-free housing; retired couples in which one partner's health is precarious; aging individuals seeking supported independence with a wide range of medical and housekeeping services.

Earlier generations of older people stayed at home until they died or were put into a nursing home. Now, many choose some sort of communal living for retirement because there are so many new options. With pensions, social security, and the inflation of recent decades boosting the equity they have in their homes, people of all but the lowest income level are able to afford some type of traditional community living.

Traditional Housing Options for
Low-income Midlife and Older People

*Federally Subsidized
Low-Rent Apartments*

The first public-housing project developed by the American government for older people was built in San Antonio, Texas, in the sixties. This project was to be the start of a renaissance period in federally subsidized housing for the aged. More often than not, the housing was built for the frail and dependent older person. However, some healthy low-income people were fortunate enough to benefit from such government housing.

My eighty-four-year-old aunt is an occupant of public housing. She says:

After forty-seven years in a gradually deteriorating apartment in the city, I am living in a lovely, spacious apartment. It's a public-housing project for senior citizens, and I was one of the first chosen in a lottery (with 800 others still on a waiting list). I have three and a half bright, sunny rooms with an outside porch. My total rental cost is seventy-two dollars a month. My neighbors and I have a van that takes us to the nearby village to shop once a week, and we have a central building for our many recreational programs. One neighbor drives me to the Retired Senior Volunteer Program twice a week, where I type and regularly call on other homebound seniors. I feel secure. There are buzzers in every room in case I need help, and a round-the-clock manager. I've never been happier.

A middle-aged friend tells much the same story about her mother:

My seventy-seven-year-old mother is living in a state-subsidized public-housing project in Brooklyn. Among twenty buildings, three are set aside for seniors. These three contain 200 apartments—each individual and lovely. This arrangement is not only important to my mother but to my siblings and me. Mom is able

117

to maintain her own independence (she is determined not to live with any of us), and yet she is not alone. Someone will always be there when she needs help—either one of her new friends or the building manager. She has an arrangement with a friend across the court. Shades are pulled down when each woman goes to bed and pulled up by eight o'clock the next morning. Any variance from this safety routine is followed by a phone call to family members and/or a call for the manager.

Although government-funded public housing has been very successful, during the Reagan years the country experienced a drastic reduction in federally subsidized housing for the low-income elderly.

Recycled Schools: Coming Home to the Classroom

Adaptive reuse of vacant property to meet the growing need for housing is occurring in every state in the country. A convent in Chicago became shared housing for the elderly; a seminary in Ohio is now a retirement community; an abandoned hospital in New Hampshire was renovated to become ninety-four units of subsidized congregate housing, as did a college dormitory in Boston.

As the population of young people decreases and that of older people grows, more and more schools are becoming available for conversion housing—and much of that for midlife and older people.

A typical old-fashioned classroom produces generous one-bedroom apartments with large windows and high ceilings. To those able to remain in a familiar community setting, recycling is well worth the effort.

Chester Commons

Chester Commons is a former high school and library in the small town of Chester, Massachusetts. Combining the memories of the past with the convenience of today's modern apartment living, each of the fifteen two- and three-room units reflects many of the architectural details of the original school. Chester Commons is open to independent people over age fifty-five. Residents of the village of Chester are given first priority, and admission is based on income eligibility. Most people who live in "The Commons" have some sort of family or community ties.

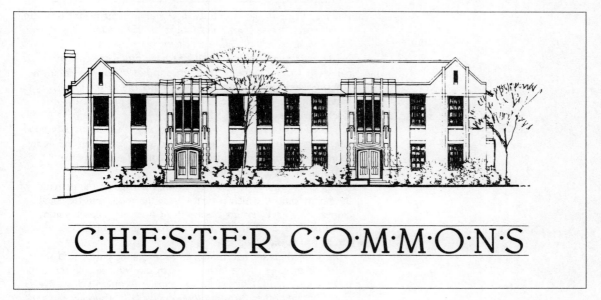

C·H·E·S·T·E·R C·O·M·M·O·N·S

Chester Commons, Chester, Massachusetts.

These subsidized apartments require that a single individual have an adjusted annual income of no more than $14,504 (or $16,576 for couples) and no more than $15,000 worth of assets. Tenants pay 25 percent of their monthly income as rent, which includes heat and hot water. The Massachusetts Chapter 707 Program pays the difference between the tenant's share and the total rent cost.

One married couple, six men, and eight women live in Chester Commons. They all must be independent and healthy, since there are the stairs to climb. There are no supportive services, with the exception of a maintenance man (living next door) who works every day and a project manager who comes by once a week.

I was given a tour of the Commons by the project manager, during which I interviewed a seventy-year-old resident, Mrs. Leoni. She is the mother of two, grandmother of seven, and recently became a great-grandmother. When Mrs. Leoni separated from her husband, she moved from their home in Connecticut "back home" to Chester and become one of the original tenants of the Commons.

For me, living in my new town-house apartment meant returning to my roots. I was born and brought up in Chester. One of the men I went to school with many long years ago, as well as a neighbor of mine when my children were little, has chosen to live here too. I came home because my son has a summer cabin in Chester, and my daughter and her family are in the process of building a new home here. This brings them into town from Rochester almost every weekend.

I have lots of room for overnight or weekend guests. My good-size bedroom is upstairs, and I have a studio couch in the living room. I have dinner with two of my cousins and their family, who live in town, every week.

My days are busy. Many of us are involved in the activities of the senior center, which is right across the road, and the local church. We have regular check-ups at a nearby health center, and I drive to a town several miles away to see my personal doctor and to go shopping.

At Christmas we had an open-house eggnog party, and some of us ate together at the picnic table in our yard during the summer. I don't think I would be so happy if I couldn't drive my car. The only other transportation available is a weekly bus that can be arranged for by appointment, but only for medical visits and necessary shopping.

*Mobile Homes:
The Least Expensive
Housing Around*

Mobile homes are becoming increasingly popular among midlife and older people. There are about four million mobile homes in this country, with eight-and-a-half million people living in them. More than half of these people are retired and are representative of the white working-class population.

Mobile homes, the least expensive form of private home ownership, offer a reasonably low-cost housing alternative for retired women and men, with a median price of $30,000 for a new home and less for a used one. Most mobile homes are sold and financed with land included for $34,000 to $62,000. Monthly fees may range from $60 to $600 and include a lot, rent, water, garbage pickup, and use of the recreational facilities.

"Closed" mobile-home parks require that new homes be purchased from the developer, usually at higher prices than at independent dealers. "Open" parks allow residents to move in with their own mobile homes (although some parks will not allow homes that are older than five years). Mobile home values depreciate, unlike permanent homes, which increase in value.

The homes can be large and quite luxurious. Many include appliances and wall-to-wall carpeting. The typical size is fourteen feet wide and sixty-nine feet long. Since many are made of wood (instead of metal), they have been renamed "manufactured homes." Most mobile-home parks are found in states with mild climates, such as Arizona, California, and Florida, and usually in suburban areas. Trailer parks often have paved streets, green lawns, swimming pools, and other amenities.

People wishing to experience this kind of life-style are advised to rent a mobile home and use it for several weeks' vacation before buying. For many people, the space in a mobile home is too limited, and a trailer park lacks privacy. Most trailer parks are located in isolated areas away from shopping, police and fire protection, and medical care. A car is a virtual necessity. Some parks are very restrictive, prohibiting pets, children, and visitors who stay more than a week.

Movable Trailers

Movable trailers satisfy many older people's desire to travel. One eighty-three-year-old single woman has traveled in her large, self-contained Winnebago to every state in the union and Canada since her retirement twenty years ago. It has become an enjoyable way of life for her.

(Readers interested in mobile homes can write to the Manufactured Housing Institute, 1745 Jefferson Davis Highway, Suite 511, Arlington, Virginia 22202.)

A Retirement Community That Welcomes Religious Women

At a recent gerontology conference, I asked a lecturing Catholic nun where retired nuns could live. She sent me information about the Rocky Creek Retirement Village, which is now home to lay people, as well as to eighteen sisters from nine different congregations.

The village is funded by a unique blend of federal, state, and local programs, making it affordable housing for low- and moderate-income seniors. A flat monthly rental fee is charged (ranging from $555 to $650), with no entry fee or long-term lease required. Two meals are served each day, and residents have all of the amenities of a full-service retirement community.

According to one of the sisters in residence, "Retired sisters with their diversified talents and education have no problem finding a ministry here. We have broadened our opportunities for ministry by our loving concern and service to both staff and residents."

(Interested readers can contact Rocky Creek Village, 8606 Boulder Court, Tampa, Florida 33615; 1-800-289-3388.)

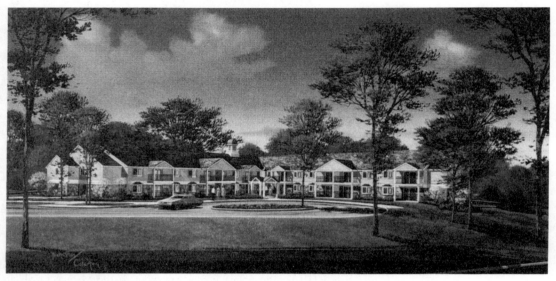

Orchard View, Carroll, Iowa.

Traditional Housing Options for Middle-income Americans

Quality Living at an Affordable Retirement Community

In recommending retirement communities, the *New York Times* suggested the beautiful state of Iowa, so I traveled to the Orchard View community in Carroll, Iowa, to see for myself.

Driving into Orchard View, I was sure I had the wrong address. It looked like a glamorous condo, with as many younger people as older coming in and out. This former site of an apple orchard had flowers and trees surrounding lounge chairs and umbrella tables. Orchard View is in west-central Iowa, two hours from the city of Des Moines and close to a large junior college.

People come to check out Orchard View from all over the country—Alaska, California, Tennessee, Kansas, and Washington, D.C. About half the residents, however, come from the surrounding towns or have a son or daughter living in the area. Fifty-five people (age sixty-four through ninety-two) live independently in this community, which advertises a minimum age of fifty. Half of them are couples, it seems, and half singles. If residents become ill, they have direct access to St. Anthony's Hospital and Nursing Home, right up the hill.

Orchard View was built for middle-income people, many of whom have recently sold their own homes. The monthly rent for a spacious one-bedroom apartment is $550. A luxurious three-bedroom apartment with a formal dining room, large walk-in closets, and a balcony rents for $800. These fees are possible because of cooperative funding from the city of Carroll and a nearby Franciscan order. This is a nonprofit community, which keeps funneling profits back into better services for the people who live there.

Rent includes all utilities and maintenance and use of private garden space, transportation, a fully equipped workroom, and exercise and game rooms. There are lovely, small lounge-rooms on each floor for an extra flow of visiting friends or relatives. Although each person can cook his/her own meals in his/her apartment, residents can choose to eat, for a reasonable cost, in the spacious community dining room. A small, private dining room is available for entertaining guests, and guest rooms are available for fifteen dollars a night.

An Orchard View couple in their early seventies that I interviewed had recently sold their large home and appeared very pleased with their new life-style.

We were delighted to divest ourselves of all but a few prized possessions while we were still together and healthy. Now I work one or two days a week as a consultant in a large investment corporation, and we love having time to participate in all of the activities here. Believe it or not, we pay less here than we did living in our own home with all of its maintenance and taxes.

123

*And yet, what price could we put on living here, where we are
so happy?*

*Our children and grandchildren live close by, but we don't
have to depend on them. We have become an incredible community in less than a year. It's our feeling that our health has improved since we've lived here—perhaps because we've been able
to leave so many responsibilities behind, have a lot of friends
here, and are more likely to exercise. One of our friends cycles
at least fifty miles a week.*

Gwen, a widow, tried staying in her family condo for
two years after her husband's death. She said:

*I was too lonely. It is hard to meet new people when you see
them only in the garage or at the dumpster! I missed, most of
all, a male viewpoint of the world. Just to hear voices, I kept my
TV on all of the time.*

*I wanted to settle somewhere else while I was still able to
make my own decisions. I'm really happy now. The people are
very nice. If you are lonesome here it's your own fault. I am
actively involved in my church, which is nearby, and I play
bridge and socialize a lot.*

As another resident put it, "I think we have one of the nicest,
most elegant, respectful, and affordable retirement communities in
the country."

(Interested readers can contact Orchard View, Carroll, Iowa 51401; 712-792-
3581.)

*Retirees Head for College
Towns*

As students head back to campus, they may find their newest neighbors are retirees. A growing trend, especially in the Northeast and
the Carolinas, is the resettling of retirees in college towns. Many
move back to the sites of the colleges they attended in their youth,
to recapture that special sense of belonging.

This is a relatively new group of middle- to upper-income
retirees, who are looking for intellectual stimulation. With the
college-age population declining and the fifty-plus population rising,
colleges realize they have much to gain by opening their programs

to older people. Housing is often reasonably priced, and the health services in college areas are excellent. Some retired professors volunteer to lecture or teach part-time, thereby enriching the educational climate. According to one retired couple:

Living near the campus is great. What we especially wanted was a place that offered a wide choice of cultural events as well as good shops and restaurants—and a college town was perfect. We believe that as long as you have intellectual curiosity, you should use it and stay young. I use the university library all the time, and we attend concerts, lectures, movies, theater, ballet, opera, and athletic events on campus. In fact, we have to be careful of becoming too busy. We enjoy younger people and wanted to avoid the golf and tennis communities that are basically for retired people. For the most part, we can count on our neighbors being more interesting than they might be in a customary retirement village.

Clemson Downs, in Clemson, South Carolina, was one of the first retirement villages to take advantage of a college setting. The complex of ninety-five apartments, a skilled nursing home, and communal dining facilities has drawn many retired businesspeople who attended Clemson years ago, as well as retired professors.

Syracuse University in upstate New York has an intergenerational-living project. Connecting high-rise buildings on the campus house 400 older people and 750 graduate students and their families. The dining hall, library, and activity areas are shared.

Duke University in Durham, North Carolina, has long sponsored the Duke Institute for Learning and Retirement. For a small fee, people over fifty who live in the area are entitled to take courses at the college, use the university pool, and are given discounts on plays and concerts.

Traditional Housing Options for Financially Well-off Americans

Housing for the affluent elderly has been a long-overlooked market enterprise, which the private-business sector has only recently begun to take advantage of. Despite the sluggish housing market and the slowdown of new housing construction, one area of real estate has experienced a sudden increase. The number of retirement and life-care communities is rapidly growing. The graying of America may be a sociological phenomenon to some, but to others it's a new housing market.

Private developers are not the only group looking at housing for older people. Churches and fraternal organizations also recognize the need for this type of community and are seeking to meet this need. The Episcopal Diocese in Connecticut is developing a 250-unit complex, and the state's Masonic Charity Foundation continues to expand Ashlar Village in Wallingford. Although rents are high (ranging from $1,850 to $2,245), this village has a waiting list of 900 people.

Adult Retirement/Leisure Communities

Many older Americans with middle or high incomes are moving to the retirement/leisure communities that are springing up across the country. After years of work, many women and men want to enjoy the recreation and leisure opportunities this type of housing provides, often in a country-club atmosphere.

Most people seek information and make plans concerning retirement communities before a change is forced upon them by circumstances—when they are still in control. Usually, married couples move into these communities after they retire and remain there after they have been widowed. Nowhere is the longevity of women over men so starkly revealed as in a retirement community, with women outnumbering men 170 to 30.

To some people in the sixty-five-plus age group, community may mean selling their home and moving to a retirement village that has comforts they never dreamed of in their working years—housekeeping services, social activities, or a swimming pool.

Moving into a group-living situation may seem like sacrificing independence, but, such a decision—made when people feel in control of their choices—tends to help them live longer and healthier lives.

Although most people base their decision to move into a retirement community on finances, health services, or ease of maintenance, they all have an underlying theme. They are looking for a life-style in which they can keep their independence.

Where Are the Retirement Villages Located?

Although early retirement villages were concentrated in the warmer climates of the South and West, developers soon recognized that many people over fifty wanted to live near their families, as well as in or near an urban environment. Within the last few years, we have witnessed what has been labeled by gerontologists as a "reverse migration," with large numbers of retirees returning to the north from Florida, Arizona, and South Carolina.

Connecticut, which is typical of other states in the Northeast, has several flourishing retirement communities for financially well-off older people. They range from those for the able-bodied to more elaborate "continuing care" or "life care" centers.

A luxury hotel in Stamford has been converted into a luxury apartment complex for the elderly, with monthly rentals ranging from $1,645 to $3,995, which covers rent, meals, and activities. Connecticut Blue Cross/Blue Shield has entered the real-estate business for the first time with a 200-resident retirement community in Hamden, built within a larger residential community for people of all ages. Condominiums here sell for $100,000 to $250,000.

Why, or Why Not, Live in a Retirement Community?

A continuing source of controversy regarding retirement communities is that they are characterized primarily by one age group. Most require that one member of each couple be age fifty or older, and children under eighteen are not allowed.

However, some people find that age-segregated residential communities enhance their participation in and enjoyment of social activity. They enjoy a heightened sense of personal security—and most important of all, a feeling of complete independence. Residents have their own rooms and baths; they eat and sleep, come and go, without having to consider someone else's likes or dislikes.

In her eighties, Gertrude Levine, who has worked for almost a decade with me on the *Hot Flash* newsletter board, expresses these thoughts on retirement-community living:

When my husband and I decided to retire, we felt that a move to a condominium in a retirement village would be the best choice for us. We have now lived in our home in this village for thirteen years and have never regretted our decision.

Our particular complex has five hundred families, who vary in age from forty-eight and up, coming from all walks of life. When we first moved in, there were fewer families, and it was very easy to get acquainted at the clubhouse and the swimming pool. Neighbors are warm and friendly but not intrusive, which made us feel welcome. Activities are plentiful for those who want to take part. The tendency is to get too involved.

There are certain restrictions in this life-style. Although you own your home, the area surrounding it is community property regulated by the rules set up by the town, the builder, and the people who are either elected or hired by the homeowners to run the condominium. For the most part, requests are reasonable and in no way interfere with the full enjoyment of your home.

The most wonderful aspect of this life-style is the caring people around us. If someone has a misfortune, not only do family and close friends respond, but also those who are just acquaintances. There is always someone to offer assistance. No one ever feels at a loss or alone. There is a great sense of security. However, your privacy is always respected. When you buy a condominium in a retirement village, you are not only buying a house, you are buying a way of life.

Some couples living in retirement communities, however, feel too separated from the wider community and from important life concerns and interests. Sometimes, one spouse is delighted with the environment of a retirement community, whereas the other feels they will "wither away and die" if they remain there.

This was the frustration of one couple I interviewed, Elisabeth and George Seefeld, who had lived almost two years in a South Carolina retirement community of three hundred homes and apartments. George, an eighty-year-old retired lawyer, says this of his experience:

I have found the level of people I like here. I admire the people of my own age. They are accomplished, and we can talk freely. I fraternize with several men in the community. There is lots of socializing, especially around cocktail parties. I have my music *and my gardening. My wife and I traveled a lot—with a scheme to visit all the great civilizations of the world—and we have done so. Now I have the pleasure of sitting down and reading about them. The climate here in South Carolina is the best thing. It's pleasantly cool in the winter; the ice and snow of Massachusetts were very wearing. I could be happy here for the rest of my life, but Elisabeth isn't. We've been married thirty-five years, and we can't separate now!*

Elisabeth, a seventy-three-year-old retired office manager, has a different story to tell.

I don't know why I agreed to move here. George wanted to terribly—he couldn't do all the work in our house in Massachusetts anymore. I can't stand it. I have no interest in doing things with all these old people. They keep asking if we play bridge. We don't, and I find it boring. I feel as though I've been moved from my lifeline—from any useful role in life. In fact, in the beginning, I was so depressed that I was ready to throw it all in. What has made it more bearable is my volunteer job two afternoons a week at a nearby university. At least I feel I'm doing something, not wasting my time. In the summers when we go back to Massachusetts, I immediately get over my feelings of gloom and doom. I think we all have a right to find an environment we feel good in or stimulated by. I fantasize about moving back north. I think that independent living is best—not being tied down to a small community in which you feel obligated to take part.

For this couple, the important thing to know is that there are many other options that they can afford—from a more active community to an urban intergenerational setting.

Traditional Retirement Communities for People Who Share Common Interests

Retirement Communities Designed Around a Person's Former Profession

Retirement communities for people who shared similar careers before retirement have also been successful. Some thriving examples include:

- York States, a New York State teachers' retirement center in Syracuse. This two-story housing development is run by the state retired teachers' association

- The Film Industry Retirement Community, in Woodland Hills, California, is a large residential community with fifty-four cottages on forty-one acres. It has 275 residents (their average age is eighty-two) who have retired from different positions in the movie industry. A hospital and health-care facility are on the premises. Says one resident, "It means a lot when you get old to be with people who understand the magic of the movies. We don't have to search for topics of conversation, because we all love show business."

- Sunset Hall, in downtown Los Angeles, was established by the Unitarian Church in 1924 as a retirement home for social and political activists. Residents support one another's decision to remain politically active. One says, "We're not wallowing in resignation here but fighting for our rights."

Retirement Villages Sponsored by Religious Organizations

A Quaker Community

Rose, an eighty-year-old friend, wrote to me about the Quaker-run retirement home she and her husband had moved to. After searching the country for just the right place to live, they found what they were looking for in Newtown, Pennsylvania.

> For us, this is perfect. So much is offered to us: protection, good food and services, stimulating activities and cultural happenings in nearby communities. No more planning and preparing meals if we don't want to. No more shoveling snow, mowing grass, fertilizing, weeding, or raking unless we want to volunteer to do it. No more calling the plumber, waiting all day for the refrigerator man, taking care of the heater, dickering with all kinds of service people. You'll have to come and experience for yourself the warm spirit that dwells among us.

And so my husband and I did! Friends Village is located in a rural area near Trenton, New Jersey, about thirty miles from Philadelphia. The village has forty-four living units—studio apartments, one- and two-bedroom units, and nonhousekeeping units.

We had dinner in a sunny dining room, with nicely dressed men and women. The conversation was lively and stimulating. Because it is a Quaker community, Friends Village not only met Rose's and her husband's physical needs, but their spiritual needs as well.

A second planned and supportive Friends Community has been built in Easton, Massachusetts, for people of all ages. It is based on the Quaker belief in peace and nonviolence. Skilled medical and nursing care is available in the nearby neighborhood. This community has 160 solar-heated townhouses, organized for legal purposes as a condominium.

(Interested readers can contact Friends Village, 331 Lower Dolington Road, Newtown, Pennsylvania 18940 or Friends Community, Lincoln Street, North Easton, Massachusetts 02356.)

An Active Community of Retired Church Professionals

Friends of mine living in San Francisco have put their name on the very long reservation list (it takes several years to gain admittance) of a retirement residence called Pilgrim Place. This is a religious and cultural center of 325 retired church professionals who have completed twenty years of Christian employment. Residents come from nearly every state and forty-five other countries of the world. Pilgrim Place, located on thirty-three acres in the college town of Claremont, California, has ten central buildings and 177 individual homes and apartments.

Admission is offered only to those between the ages of sixty-five and seventy-five who meet basic health requirements. Special consideration is given to career missionaries, members of minority groups, those willing to enter at an earlier age, and those associated with the United Church of Christ. However, the residence is ecumenical, with at least a dozen other denominations, the YMCA, and the YWCA well represented.

A proportional entrance fee of 9 percent of an applicant's net assets is charged. Residents pay monthly rent, established at less than comparable commercial rates; a monthly residential fee, which includes maintenance of all common buildings (no more than a quarter of residents' monthly incomes); and meal charges for the family-style noontime meal. No one is turned away for lack of funds, since many religious workers bring limited resources to their retirement. Although Pilgrim Place does not offer guaranteed life care, an assisted level of living is available for those who require it, and a third level of care is available in the nearby Health Services Center, a fifty-nine-bed facility offering long-term nursing care.

(Interested readers can contact Pilgrim Place, 660 Avery Road, Claremont, California 91711; 714-621-9581.)

Continuing-Care/Life-Care Communities

Continuing-care communities, a fast growing segment of the retirement-housing market, are the luxury option in group housing for seniors.

Historically connected with religious organizations and fraternal groups, continuing-care housing has existed in some form since the 1800s. In the last decade, a sluggish housing market and a dramatic increase in the number of affluent older people in this country has brought private developers and investors by the droves into continuing-care, or life-care centers for older people.

Continuing-care communities offer freedom from worries about home maintenance and security, new friends and experiences, and the security of knowing health needs will be attended to.

What's the Difference Between a Retirement Village and a Continuing-Care/Life-Care Community?

The major difference between retirement villages and life-care communities is that residents of life-care communities sign a contract in which they are guaranteed housing and other services such as meals, transportation, and health care for the rest of their lives, regardless of how their needs change over time.

Basically, couples or individuals make one very substantial initial payment, and substantial monthly payments—securing an attractive, safe place to live, in an age-segregated community, with a full range of services—for life.

Entrance fees are often called "endowments." What is being purchased is the promise of care for the rest of one's life. Residents of continuing-care retirement communities (CCRCs) seldom own their homes. People choose life-care communities primarily for access to health care and security—and only partly for social or community reasons.

Three Continuing-Care Plans

A typical CCRC comprises a large piece of land with independent living units and a nursing facility. CCRCs are designed for independent older people in reasonably good health—who want to buy peace of mind for their remaining years. There are three classifications of continuing-care plans, with nursing care the most important variable.

The All-Inclusive or Full Plan includes housing, residential and health care services, and unlimited full nursing care, if eventually needed, for about the same monthly fee paid to live independently.

The Fee-for-Service Plan (or the "unbundling" of services) is becoming more common. An entrance fee may or may not be charged. Residents may be guaranteed access to a nursing care facility, but will have to pay for such care at whatever the going rate is when they need it.

The Modified Plan falls somewhere in between the first two, providing a few days of free nursing care each year. Some facilities have an intermediate level of care—an assisted living unit where frail persons have their own room, but meals are provided and help is available as needed with bathing, medication, dressing, and other chores.

In effect, CCRC residents pool their risks with other residents. Those who stay healthy for the rest of their lives may be paying more than the cost of the services they receive. And yet, those who develop long-term disabilities that require medical care, may pay much less for that care than they otherwise would. However, the end result for all residents is insurance against long-term catastrophic medical costs.

Costs

Entrance fees range anywhere from $40,000 to $150,000—and monthly fees from $500 to $2,500. Nationwide the median entrance fee for a one-bedroom unit is $45,300, and the median monthly fee is $715. For many people, selling the home they have been living in provides much or all of the entrance fee.

The regular monthly fee covers housing, utilities, property maintenance, taxes, and insurance. It is common for CCRCs to provide such services as housekeeping, laundry, some or all meals, counseling, medical services, transportation around town, social, recreational, and religious activities. Each community provides a different range of services. The facility is quite likely to have a library, beauty and barber shops, exercise equipment, and classes. It's less likely to offer a swimming pool, garden plots, cable-TV hookups, garage parking, and the use of a guest apartment.

One of the myths about continuing-care communities is that you give them all your money, and you never get it back, and this may have been true of the earlier life-care centers. Today a contract will specify whether or not any of the entrance fee will be refunded to you or your estate when you move or die. Two-thirds of all continuing-care retirement communities have a "declining refund" policy under which less is refunded the longer you live there. Some facilities refund nothing after an initial trial period. Others may guarantee the refund of most of the fee no matter how long you live there.

Despite the many advantages of continuing-care communities, there is uncertainty about the impact of inflation and rising medical costs on future expenses. Monthly fees, because they cover operating expenses, will need to be adjusted to keep pace with the economy. Since the investment required by a CCRC resident often represents a substantial piece of total personal assets, residents want to know their investment is safe. Thirty-one states have now enacted legislation regulating CCRCs, and a number of other states are considering such legislation to avoid fraudulent practices or marketing misrepresentation.

A Rapidly Growing Industry

Continuing-care communities are a rapidly growing industry in this country. Today, there are more than 700 facilities in the United States, with an expectation of 1,500 by the end of the century. An estimated 250,000 older people have chosen to live in such communities (less than 1 percent of all older people). The selling of residences in life-care communities has proven to be as profitable as the selling of condominiums.

Although developers have a lot of respect for this potential housing market, they use some rather irreverent labels among themselves to describe the three groups of elderly which are attracted to this type of housing.

- Early retirees, active and healthy, interested in travel, new experiences, and independent living are referred to as "go-go's."
- Older retirees who remain active, but may be widowed or in need of some help are called "slow-go's."
- The frail elderly, still partially independent but unable to manage the tasks of daily living without assistance, are called "no-go's."

Hotel Chains are Plunging Into the Life-Care Field

One-third of all life care facilities are operated for profit by large private developers such as the Hyatt Hotels and the Marriott Corporation.

Marriott Senior Living Services is a new subsidiary of Marriott with projects designed for the life-care market. When I spoke to him, the vice-president said, "Of the current sixty-five-plus American market, 81 percent own their own home, 64 percent without a mortgage. Financially, more are in good shape than are struggling." It is this middle-income-and-above bracket of older people that the hotel chains have aggressively moved in to service.

Marriott's congregate-care business has two parts: *independent full service,* and *catered living* for those needing more assistance. Residents who age and grow frail can move through the various levels of care.

Most hotel-sponsored continuing-care communities are far from the Sun Belt, since research has shown that 92 percent of retired people want to remain near their home area. The communities are being built near such cities as Philadelphia, Arlington, and Washington, D.C.

Interested people are advised to visit as many communities as possible, compare fees and services, and chose the one best suited to their needs and life-style. Plan to spend a few days or a week in guest accommodations, or sublet an apartment for a short time to get a feel for the community, and the people you might be sharing your life with. Some people begin to visit life-care communities in their early seventies—putting down an initial application deposit (in the neighborhood of $1,000) in the community of their choice. Waiting lists can be as long as six or seven years.

Guidelines for Those Considering a Continuing-Care Community

1. Is the community financially sound? Each CCRC should be willing to provide a prospective resident with information about the community's financial condition, which you may wish to have a lawyer or financial advisor examine.

2. Read your continuing-care contract and other documents carefully, and review them with a competent advisor, attorney, or banker (one who is not associated with the facility), in order to know realistically what to expect from your CCRC.

3. Be fully aware of the contract's duration, and the policy for refunds or adjustments in fees if you decide to leave the community, or at the time of your death.

4. Learn under what circumstances monthly fees will increase. If they increase with inflation, ask to what extent.

5. Ask whether or not your state has laws protecting retirement home residents from fraud and financial collapse. For example, Pennsylvania has established strong laws—and, to date, New York State prohibits combining hotel residency with health care in one facility.

6. Ask what would happen if for any reason you ever became unable to pay the monthly charges.

7. If you are transferred to the facility's nursing care section, how long will your living unit remain yours? What decision making policy exists to handle such situations?

8. Know the specifics of the health care offered. What medical insurance coverage will you be required to carry? Is dental, vision, and hearing care covered in the contract? What about medications? Is there a limit on inpatient or outpatient care—and what about rehabilitative services? Check the status of the license of the health care agency.

9. What extra fees will be charged—and how much? Does your regular fee cover such additional features as the swimming pool, trips and excursions, hairdressing, craft classes?

10. Find out the extent of resident participation in decision making.

Some Personal Accounts

The eighty-nine-year-old grandmother of a friend told the following story about her continuing-care retirement community in Pennsylvania.

EVELYN HALE

In 1976, after twenty-five years of living in Connecticut (first in a circa 1740 farmhouse, then in a dream house on our own wildlife preserve, and finally in a condominium), the time came when my husband, and then I, decided to stop driving. This decision, in turn, meant that we would have to look into new living arrangements.

Although our daughter and son-in-law suggested building an apartment for us in the garden of their suburban home, we thought we should look into retirement communities first. We knew of many, where our friends lived, but none suited our needs. We wanted to live in the country on a hilly terrain.

Hearing of our quest, a neighbor loaned us a brochure which described a new life-care community in a rural area near Doylestown, Pennsylvania. It was on a lake, near wildlife preserves, and was 300 feet above sea level. After a visit to look it over, we decided that this was the place for us. We applied for membership, had our physicals, and were accepted.

This proved to be the wisest decision we ever made. We found a place where all our needs are met—we have a spacious apartment with a view, a medical center that provides complete care, proximity to a fine hospital, nourishing and attractively served meals, twenty-four-hour security, transportation for shopping, and friendly, congenial people. There is a pervading air of sincere caring by both staff and members.

The monthly fee is based on the type of apartment, the age and health of the applicant, and the amount of the down payment. Although this life-care community is rather costly, we were pleased to learn that the IRS allows a generous percentage of the monthly fee as a medical deduction.

Our First Year

Our first year was a glamorous experience. We participated in all activities—lectures, concerts, trips, and sports. We took long walks and danced at parties and made many good friends. In 1977, after my husband had surgery for a broken hip, our activities were seriously curtailed. But because we were living in a life-care community, he was able to return home from the on-site medical center. With the aid of a walker, he stayed with me in the apartment for three years before it became necessary for him to have skilled nursing care in the medical center. I feel that he received more loving care there than he would have received in the usual nursing home.

When my husband died, I was fortunate to have the support of warm friends. Because many of them have known the pain of bereavement, they were able to help me greatly during a very sad time.

Now, at eighty-nine, I walk about a mile a day using a cane as a safety measure. The days are never long enough to accomplish all I plan—but each day I give thanks for having found a beautiful place to live and good friends to share it with.

Eighty-one-year-old Ann Herrick is a former teacher who lives in a continuing-care community just outside of the city of Bridgeport,

Connecticut. She is the mother of two sons and has five adult grandchildren. Widowed for fifteen years, she has a master's degree, in Greek and Latin, from Columbia University and was a teacher until age seventy-six.

My husband and I visited with her in a beautiful high-rise apartment building, surrounded by twelve acres of lovely gardens. The community, called Thirty Thirty Park (after its address), was founded in 1968 under the sponsorship of the Council of Churches of Greater Bridgeport. Residents pay a one-time continuing-care fee, based on the size and location of the apartment they select (ranging from $27,000 for a studio to $114,500 for a three room)—and a monthly fee from $891 to $1,964. Each person owns their own apartment, and is provided with three meals a day, heat, air conditioning, weekly cleaning services, flat laundry, telephone, security, recreational facilities, and access to the health center. To live here, people must be sixty-two or over, with no upper age limit. The oldest resident is one hundred years old.

We joined Ann and several good friends for a delicious lunch in a light and sunny dining room. Later, settled in her cozy apartment, she told us the following story:

ANN HERRICK

I'd visited several other life-care communities outside of Philadelphia, where I had one or two friends—and they each said, "Ann, you'd love it here." But for me that would mean moving away from my large network of social and professional friends and family. I knew about Thirty Thirty from the day of its inception, and had visited friends here often.

After my husband's death, I lived alone for several years—constantly worrying about the leak in the chimney, or the driveway that needed repair. What brought it all to a head was the day I fell over my dog and broke my leg. It took a while for someone to find me, and then I wasn't able to stay alone with my ankle-to-hip cast. For me, the decision was clear—"Thirty Thirty here I come!" Fortunately my name had been on the waiting list, so I had to wait less than a year to move in.

For a woman alone, a one-bedroom apartment is just the right size. I paid $55,000 for my apartment five years ago and now it's worth $100,000—and my monthly rent is $1,200. I have all of my own furniture, plants, and books. I pay extra for my medical care, which is available in a one-hundred-bed health wing.

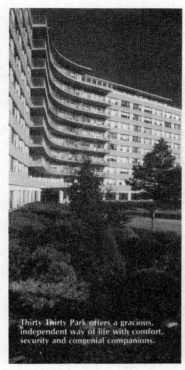

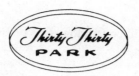

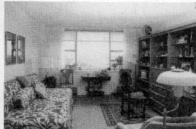

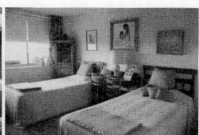

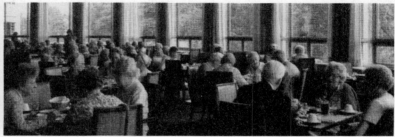

Thirty Thirty Park offers a gracious, independent way of life with comfort, security and congenial companions.

Thirty Thirty Park, Bridgeport, Connecticut.

A Typical Day

Every morning when I wake up, I call the office to let them know I'm "just fine." Each apartment has a small kitchenette, so I rarely go down to breakfast. I love to just luxuriate here in my room—listening to the seven o'clock news, reading the New York Times while I have toast, juice, and coffee. Later in the morning there's always a committee meeting, or my writers group. I either eat lunch in the dining room or make a sandwich to eat on my little balcony. In the afternoons I go for walks, shopping, have a friend in for tea, read, or go visit my friends in nearby Westport. I always have dinner in the dining room with my friends, watch the MacNeil/Lehrer news, or an old movie, or play bridge. Some evenings we have a special concert, dance performance, or lecture. Many people go into the Saturday afternoon opera in New York City, or to the theater.

If I were to become sick I would go to the health center for a

Who Might Enjoy Living at Thirty Thirty?

few days, and then come back. If I needed daily care I would have to give up my apartment and live there.

When you ask me who might like to live here, I would say upper middle-class, professional people. Most of us have had quite vivid careers. A college background helps. Couples just love it, as do many of us who are now single. Interestingly enough, there are several pairs of sisters living here.

I feel I am in control of my own life here—as much as when I lived in my own home. I come and go without anyone questioning me, and leave my apartment for long vacations. My son just visited from Hawaii, and spent a week in one of our guest rooms. I've found six good friends with somewhat similar backgrounds. We find each other stimulating and laugh at the same jokes. One of the wonderful things about this place is the caring of people—the neighborly feelings. Thirty Thirty is just the right place for me now, and I am very happy with my life.

(Interested readers can contact Thirty Thirty Park, 3030 Park Avenue, Bridgeport, Connecticut 06604; 203-374-5611.)

Chapter Seven

Living Near Family

The late Margaret Mead maintained that societies were more stable when families were intergenerational. Why, then, is a family life-style so frowned upon? Sometimes it is impossible or undesirable to share housing with family members, because there simply is no room or their life-style makes this too difficult. But living close by one's family *can* work, as the following stories illustrate.

Living on the Property of an Adult Child

ECHO (Elder Cottage Housing Opportunity) Homes or elder cottages are prefabricated houses transported by truck to the side or rear yard of an adult child or other family member. They usually are quite lovely, with one or two bedrooms, a living room, and a kitchen and bath. They also include a heater and washer and dryer. An ECHO home has enormous potential as a low-cost alternative housing model for many people. A well-built unit can be installed for about $18,000, and the proximity of the home makes it possible for each family to pursue their own lives and yet maintain close contacts through informal drop-in visits and shared meals.

ECHO housing is about giving and getting support.

Grandparents can give more attention to young children when their parents are absent, and adult children can help out with shopping and strenuous household chores. All involved may feel a greater sense of security with ECHO housing. ECHO housing obviously is an ingenious solution to the growing problem adult children face in parental care-giving.

Patterned after the Australian Granny Flat Program, the first American elder cottage was built near Lebanon, Pennsylvania, in the early eighties, costing $20,000. However, this housing program has been slow to develop in America, because of strict local zoning laws.

"Outbuildings," the original name for this type of housing, have a long tradition in America. Small towns all over the country have two homes sharing a lot. In some areas, however, residents who value the single-family character of a town are afraid that "temporary" ECHO housing will lower property values, spoil the looks of a residential neighborhood, remain in place forever, raise the cost of social services, and cause parking problems.

A few interested builders who have presented their cases to the town boards in Frederick County, Maryland, Colerain Township and Lancaster County, Pennsylvania, and in Tucson, Arizona, have convinced the boards to grant exemptions to their existing zoning laws "for a specific individual or individuals, with the precondition that they will be the only occupants." California has also enacted legislation encouraging elder cottages. They are setting out to prove that ECHO homes are attractive and are built for easy dismantling and moving. At present, an estimated 13 percent of all manufactured homes are located (legally or illegally) in the backyards of family and friends.

One middle-aged couple in Pennsylvania says, "We couldn't be happier with the results. It feels so much better knowing my mother is close to us. We can take care of her needs, but she still doesn't feel she is imposing on us."

An older couple living in an elder cottage near their son's land say they had always been concerned about emergencies, "but now our family is right here, just in case."

ECHO housing is an idea whose time has come, and changes in the zoning regulations in the United States are overdue. The addition of this life-style option would enrich the housing choices available to older Americans.

The Amish Community Small House or Grossdaadi Haus

ECHO housing is indeed an "echo" of an Amish housing model that has been in existence for hundreds of years. It is Amish tradition to provide care for the elderly within the family. Retirement, which occurs anywhere from age fifty to age seventy in the Amish community, involves a gradual decrease in active farming and a move to the *Grossdaadi Haus,* also referred to as the *doddy* or "small house." This respected tradition means that a married son or daughter will move into the parents' house, at the same time the older couple moves into a nearby "small house." Under the watchful eyes and advice of the older couple, the younger marrieds will take over the active farming.

A "Granny Flat" for Daughter and Family

When I first met Doris, she was in her late seventies, rapidly losing her eyesight, and living alone in a large, old stone house close to the center of a tiny town. She attended church, walked each day to the general store to pick up her mail and food (protected by the fierce barking of her little dog), was transported by friends to a few social events in the town, and was struggling with the help of large-print books to continue her avid reading. Every spring she would load my arms with lilacs from her garden.

Several months later, I noticed a lovely, small, unattached home built close to Doris's. Her daughter, son-in-law, and grandchildren had moved there to help her out. Doris's eyesight grew progressively worse—and her grandchildren grew to be teenagers, needing much more room than the tiny house allowed. A switch was arranged, a connecting room was built between the two homes, and Doris moved into the smaller house, where she lived until her death. This spring, her *daughter* loaded my arms with lilacs.

(Readers interested in ECHO housing can contact Coastal Colony Corporation, 2935 Meadow View Road, Manheim, Pennsylvania 17545.)

Living Near an Adult Child

Most older people own their own homes or apartments and choose to remain in them, even when that means living alone. This is often possible when an adult child lives nearby and can offer a strong, supportive, and loving relationship.

A colleague of mine from Boston wrote the following:

Let me pass along one idea my husband and I worked out for my mother-in-law, a widow of three decades (she is now eighty-eight). She still lives by herself in a ground-floor apartment in a building located on the same street that we live on. We rent the apartment across the hall from her and then, with her permission, sublet it for free to a young couple, usually graduate students, who provide company, interest in a new field (archeology, psychology, or religious studies), and who increasingly do the marketing, cooking, and so on. This arrangement has worked well for six years now.

Another long-term colleague suggested that I go down to Washington, D.C., to talk to Martha Landsman, a ninety-four-year-old widow who has had a similar arrangement for the past four years.

MARTHA LANDSMAN

When I first came to Washington at age seventy I lived in an old-age home. I wasn't happy there and stayed for only two months. People sat in rows and watched others come and go. I wasn't looking for that, so I "escaped." I went back to New York, sold my apartment, and then, with the help of my son, Otto, and his wife, Ruth, found this well-located apartment, where I've lived for twenty-three years. I am old, but I can still do almost everything for myself. My eyes are not very good, so I try to be very orderly so that I can find everything.

I am the last living person in my own family—and all of my old friends have died, except one who is exactly my age. I've known her since we were nineteen. She doesn't see well anymore, but she is always so pleased when I arrive for a visit.

My health is fine. I had a cancer operation in 1971 and have been kept on an even keel ever since by a good doctor and medicine. I have frequent skin cancers, which means running to the doctor's quite often. I try to live a very regular life, with a regular schedule, and take my medicines exactly the way they're prescribed.

When it seemed as though I needed some extra help to remain independent (like getting to the doctor and going shopping), my son and his wife decided to rent the apartment next door. They are professors, and they put up signs on the bulletin boards of their universities, offering a lovely rent-free apartment in exchange for helping me out. They do the first screening interview with applicants. I am not looking to be entertained or to form a social relationship. I tidy up and do a little cleaning and have a woman come in every two weeks to do heavy cleaning. I need my laundry and shopping done, and a companion for trips to the doctor and for my daily walk. I need someone to be quickly available to me if a need arises and to help out if I am not feeling well. When I need the person next door, I call them by phone or go knock on their door. I could even knock on the wall if necessary.

The first woman who came to live in the apartment next door was a graduate student who stayed two years. She is a beautiful, intelligent, and thoughtful person. I love her like a granddaughter, and she loves me. She still comes to see me every two weeks and is taking me to the theater next week.

The second woman stayed only a few weeks and then decided she wanted to get married. The person who is here now is a very nice nurse. In the beginning, she didn't seem very friendly, but now she is more relaxed, and we are getting along fine.

I have recently written two family histories—of my own family and one of my husband's. I was married when I was twenty-one (my father said I could have one dowry—for marriage or for study, and dumb as I was, I chose marriage). We had to leave Germany for England with our four children. My husband died there, and I brought my family here to America when the youngest was thirteen and the oldest not quite twenty. We lived in New York for twenty-five years.

The Importance of Family

I have a very large and very close family, which has been a continuous thread in my life. Whenever I need my children, they come. I used to have them all for dinner every Friday night, and now when they come, they bring most of the meal.

One of my sons lives close by, in Bethesda, Maryland. I live down here to be close to him. My oldest son and daughter live in California. They visit here whenever they can, and I go out every summer to spend four weeks with them. Another daughter lives in Canada and comes to see me often.

I'm Lucky to Have Reached Ninety-four

But best of all, I have a granddaughter and a great-granddaughter who live right here in Washington. The little one is just six months old and comes to visit me every week. She laughs out loud whenever she sees me. This is a gift. I have fourteen grandchildren, and fourteen great-grandchildren. Now it's my grandchildren who take pictures every three weeks and send them to me. They also send videos, which are even nicer than the pictures. I am very happy with them all and without complaint in my life. There is peace and love in this family, and I know I'm lucky to have reached the age of ninety-four.

Living in the Same House as an Adult Child

Several newsletters carried a small advertisement asking people over forty who lived in a "different" living arrangement to write to me. The following letter came from Rosann White, in Morrisville, Vermont.

> My daughter (forty-two) and I (sixty-nine) seem to fit your category. We occupy one house outside Morris-ville, in a fairly unusual arrangement.
>
> In 1981, my beloved housemate died, and I found myself living alone in a large house outside of Pittsburgh. My daughter, Val, a lawyer, was living alone in Vermont. When I visited her for Christmas, she invited me to come live with her. My life in Pittsburgh included helpful neighbors, congenial friends, and a very satisfactory church affiliation. Even though I was healthy, I realized that someday my daughter might have to care for me, and the distance between our two homes was great.
>
> Although we have always been congenial companions, there was no way I could live in her second bedroom! The thought horrified me; we have totally different life-styles—and even kitchen styles. We decided that I would pay off her mortgage in return for a half ownership in the house, and I would build a completely separate apartment on the second floor. I also bought another acre of land with a pond and a pasture for our five horses, three dogs, and four cats.
>
> I cook dinner and breakfast for us Monday through Thursday, and Val does the weekends. We go to church, sing in the choir, help entertain each other's guests, and share interesting books.

Here are Val's recent impressions:

> My mother was an unusual person—and not easy to live with. Fortunately, about most things, we agreed in basic philosophy. Back in the sixties she wrote to me: "Let us be all our lives hereafter not so much mother and daughter as friends and kinswomen." And we were.
>
> Our arrangement was made easier by the fact that my mother had enough money to make the

changes in my house that she wanted to make. She cooked for both of us 75 percent of the time—except on Fridays, when we took off from each other. We did laundry cooperatively, and she did my mending. A friend of hers warned her not to end up as my "wife," but truthfully, I don't think she minded. We would call each other's attention to spectacular sunsets, or interesting kinds of birds, or the antics of the horses in the pasture.

After she moved in with me, my mother had a lot of new experiences that I think she valued. She sang a tenor-soprano duet with me in church, went to a hot-air-balloon rally, rode our young stallion, and got the lead in *Arsenic and Old Lace* at our community theater.

I'm glad we made the choice to live together. I think she was as happy with me at this stage of her life as she would have been anywhere else. She enjoyed my comings and goings, my chatter, news of my daily life, and meeting my friends. I was there for her in her several illnesses, and I was there with her the morning she died. After her heart attack, I had to tell the doctors not to attempt resuscitation if she arrested.

I loved her. She was the best mother to me that she knew how to be, and I'm glad we shared the last four years of her life. She was only seventy when she died, and I wish she could have lived another quarter century.

Mother and Daughter Buying a Home Together: Lousiville, Kentucky

Two years ago, my good friend Kathy Bartlett moved with her company from New York to Kentucky, and lived in a third-floor apartment in Louisville. Recently she wrote the following to me:

Mother and I are nestled comfortably in our new home. There has been a whirlwind of decision and activity; twenty days ago, I received a phone call from Mother, letting me know that all was not well in her world. Ten hours later, my daughter and I walked into Mother's little house in Florida. We quickly made the decision that she would come back with us, prepared her household goods to be moved, and together took the plane back to Louisville.

Just eight days later, we closed on our new house, Mother's furnishings arrived, and we moved in.

We had part of my fifty-fifth birthday celebration that night in our cheerful, funky kitchen.

My heart is so full! To see the steady improvement in Mother's health and spirit, has been a joy that cannot be described. She is able to eat better, and her cane remains in the corner, quite forgotten. What a joy to be sent off each morning with a kiss and to return to her loving spirit. My life is so much richer. God works in mysterious ways, for even though I was in the process of buying a house, I really felt strongly that I wanted a house for more than just me. Mother and I have the "Welcome" mat out for all of you.

Living with Siblings

A recent newspaper story told of three sisters who left home to marry and raise their families. Nearly sixty years later, after their husbands had died, they returned to their quiet hometown and moved in together.

In the early stages of their widowhood, the sisters began traveling together—to Greece, Africa, and Turkey. At one point, they made a pact to live out their last years as a family—and they did. They share chores as they did when they were kids, never borrow each other's clothes, have their own bathrooms, and spend lots of time reminiscing. They succeeded in avoiding the loneliness, isolation, and depression that can come with old age.

Chapter Eight

Community Living Around the World

A European History of Community Housing Options

Community living in Europe began as early as the first decades of the nineteenth century. These communities offered easy access to services and were well suited for integrated age groups. Most were planned for old and young singles, and for married couples whose children had left home.

A history of community living in Europe is contained in the recent book by Franck and Ahrentzen, *New Households, New Housing* (New York: Van Nostrand Reinhold, 1989). The movement was based upon the idea of emancipating women from daily cooking and household chores. One of the first plans was developed when a Frenchman named Fourier proposed the formation of a cooperative society based on social units called *phalanges*. He proposed a community with 300 to 2,000 persons inhabiting a common building—with a centralized kitchen service—in which individual apartments would be complemented by a series of common rooms.

Fourier's ideas came to fruition in 1859, in collective housing for workers called *familistere*, with a central kitchen and dining room. Husbands and wives had separate rooms, and all housekeeping functions became collectivized.

At the end of the nineteenth century, the British pioneered a new type of urban residential building for affluent singles and elderly couples. These "catering flats" were similar to American apartment hotels, with self-contained suites, meals in a common dining room, and household services.

In the beginning of this century, the Danish *kollektivhus*, or collective house, was developed by Otto Fick. These apartments were kitchenless, and meals were served by dumbwaiters from a central kitchen. This idea spread to Sweden, Germany, Switzerland, Austria, and even to Russia, where they were called *dom-kommunas*. Both Denmark and Sweden have experimented extensively with communal living in the private and public sectors.

Scandinavian Communities

Sweden

Swedes have developed the most varied forms of publicly sponsored community life-styles. The drive for communal housing became a political movement, with banners reading "Communal Housing Now". In the sixties and seventies, small groups of Swedish friends shared more traditional communes by building their homes around a central kitchen. These were called "big family groups," or *storfamilj*. A group of Swedish female architects, designers, and journalists developed a small-scale, publicly financed rental model in which work would be shared, and people of all ages and social groups would mix. A newer form of multigenerational communal dwellings is called *kollektivhus*. Each household has private space and the potential for common meals, and shares communal facilities.

Denmark

Strandlund, Gentofte

In Denmark, it is illegal to operate profit-making nursing homes for elderly who desire or require assistance. Strandlund, known as a "sheltered flat," is the antithesis of a nursing home. Built with public funds, it is a housing project for the elderly, consisting of 210 units in a two-story building, with windows facing a large estate.

It is located in the town of Gentofte in western Denmark, near the southern tip of Sweden.

There are 144 subsidized rental units and 66 privately owned units (costing up to $175,000). Strandlund contains a social center, a swimming pool, and a small restaurant where hot lunches are served.

Each apartment receives a call each morning to make sure all is well. Units are connected to a round-the-clock nursing station. "Helpers" will shop, cook meals, and do laundry for those who need this assistance. When help is unnecessary, it is not pushed; self-determination and self-reliance are major goals of this community.

The Netherlands

Holland

Three years ago I met Heleen Toet of Huizen, Holland, at an international meeting. She told me about the community she lived in—Westhove, Huizen—and how happy and contented she felt living there:

I live in Bijvanck, a central women's project in Huizen. The name of the street is Westhove. As we are the only building on that street (named after a castle in the southwest of Holland), we speak of our home as "the castle Westhove." It is as large as a castle, with fifty apartments of two to five rooms. Each apartment has a kitchenette, a toilet, and a shower. Warm meals are prepared in the common kitchens (we have eight kitchen clusters). We share living rooms, washing rooms, a cafe, a library, a hobby room, and a playground for small children.

The building contains various corridors (or indoor "streets" as we call them), with apartments, kitchens, and community rooms on both sides. On my "street," I live with three people over fifty-five. Although most of the other inhabitants are younger, there is one other man and a woman over fifty-five.

Two or three times a week we have dinner together. Whoever wants to cook writes his or her name down on a list—and whoever wants to eat that meal does the same. The person who does the shopping and cooking, apportions the costs among all of us.

In addition to eating together, we meet frequently in the

kitchen, washing room, or in the garden. I grow vegetables in one part of our kitchen garden. Once a month we have a general meeting to decide on rules, cleaning, new occupants, etc. I am the chair of the occupant's committee. We have parties, holidays, and sporting games in small groups.

I very much like living in this way—not having to cook every day and always having someone around to share my troubles or joy, to repair things, or to take care of my cat and dog. When I want to be alone, I can retire to my own apartment. More and more older people in Holland are forming clusters to live together, and most clusters consist mainly of women. Even my "castle" has two times more women than men.

Heleen and her friend Mariet (a sixty-five-year-old woman who lives in her cluster) are very interested in all types of alternative life-styles. They were planning a trip and agreed to let me know if they found any interesting communities. This is their report about three groups they visited in Amsterdam.

Prinsengracht: A Living Group for Older Women

Mariet and I visited a house on one of Amsterdam's canals. The house is beautiful, and so are the apartments. It was built two years ago, between two seventeenth-century homes. We joined them in their "open table" monthly meeting.

Sixteen women (fifty to fifty-seven) each have two rooms in this house (men are not welcomed!). They have one community room with a kitchen, balcony, guest room, and washing room. Every morning, some of them have breakfast together. Apart from that, we did not get the impression that they shared many activities. However, the women of the house are individually very active. One of them was planning a trip to China to walk the "silk route" to Tibet.

WOOS, Woongroep Ouderen Oude Schans

This group of older people, age fifty-seven to eighty-seven, began living five years ago in a newly built canal house in the old center of town. The house consists of fourteen two- or three-room apartments. The tenants are women, one single man, and two couples. The house was built for people from the neighborhood. Eleven of the occupants originate from this part of the town.

They have a large community room, with a kitchen, balcony, guest room with bath, laundry, bicycle storage, and a garden. Once every two weeks they have dinner together and general meetings. They are committed to helping one another whenever necessary—even through illness or tragedy.

Spoorzicht

This house doesn't have an exclusive residency of older women, but my friend Astrid (fifty-six) has lived here for many years. Apart from her, the residents are younger people, living in two clusters of six people each. Astrid's cluster has a very nice and large living area where they take all their meals. Each person has one room of his/her own, and they share toilets and bathrooms.

The house has been renovated and is situated on the north side of the railway, on one of the so-called islands—Bickerseiland—in Amsterdam.

Continental Europe

Belgium

Joan Seacord is a sixty-seven-year-old colleague of mine who lives in Brussels, Belgium. She is the director of The Women's Organization for Equality. She told me about the community in which she and her husband live:

The house we live in has ninety-eight rooms—including sixty-four bedrooms, several lounges, an upstairs and a downstairs kitchen. It also includes a large conference room, offices and reception area, a communications room, a family dining room, a great hall that regularly seats fifty people for dinner (with candlelight and wine on Saturday night), and a sylvan courtyard garden that is a sanctuary of flowers and bird song.

At the turn of the century, this house was run by the Sisters of Divine Perseverance as a hostelry for young single women who had come to work in the city. Today it is the European center for an international development organization that is run by volunteers. My husband and I are two of those volunteers.

We share the everyday tasks of cooking and cleaning, the expenses of life, meals and celebrations, and we look forward to the Friday Night Pub. Our daily work is that of "human development" in villages and in organizations of both the first and third world. In the midst of our likenesses and differences, we are bonded to each other in a way that is beyond explanation.

When I walk in the front door at the end of a trip, people passing through the lobby and working in the nearby offices will come to greet me. There will be hugs and smiles of welcome. Someone will bring tea; someone else will take my luggage upstairs. I love living here. I'm home.

West Germany

In Munich, West Germany, older individuals who are willing to give up their large homes receive $3,000 in moving assistance, plus a smaller apartment. In 1980, 250 younger families took part in the housing exchange, saving an estimated $13 million. This is the estimated cost of constructing 250 large new units for these young families if the housing exchange did not exist.

France

France has a large elderly population and is developing an interesting array of housing options. Among these are *Edilys*, small apartment houses being constructed in central city sites. Each has about fifteen apartments with common areas and an optional food service. Residents pay monthly fees of $480–$640, plus a deposit of 24 percent of the investment cost. This guarantees the use of their unit for life, and their deposit is reimbursed whenever they leave or die.

The British Isles

England

The Abbyfield Society

The Abbyfield Society is one of the oldest known experiments in small-group housing. Formed in 1959, Abbeyfield, a national voluntary organization, provides family-type homes at low cost in England, Wales, Scotland, and Northern Ireland. Six to eight older people live in each home as a family—usually in the same city or town where they have lived previously. Most residents are women who can look after themselves (the average age is eighty-two) and most pay their own way, but supplementary benefits are available. Abbeyfield houses are often converted from large homes located in the middle of a residential area. Each person brings their own furnishings to their bed/sitting room. A housekeeper provides the noon and evening meals in a communal dining room. These homes are near transportation and shopping and offer older people both privacy and companionship.

Gifted Housing

In England, a charity organization called Help the Aged developed the concept of "Gifted Housing" to deal with the situation of large, underinhabited homes and the need for additional housing for the elderly. Homes that are donated by older people to Help the Aged are converted into rental apartments for other elderly persons. The donor and their spouse can live rent free for the rest of their lives in one of the renovated apartments. The elderly are able to live in a familiar surrounding and have companionship with other older people, and they are freed from taxes and maintenance costs.

Scotland

Findhorn

Findhorn, one of the very first spiritual communities of lay people, was established more than twenty-five years ago by Peter and Eileen Caddy and Dorothy Maclean. It is located on a twenty-three-acre caravan park on the coast of northeast Scotland and has served as an example to thousands of people seeking a new culture and way of life. From its earliest beginnings, Findhorn has pioneered methods of restoring the ecological balance and of cleaning up the air, water, soil, and food-supply pollution.

People of all ages from all over the world are drawn to Findhorn. For those who are consciously trying to make a difference in the world, it is a place to go to "anchor the spirit" and to release creative energy. More than one hundred people live in the community on a permanent basis, and short-term visitors are welcomed.

Findhorn is an educational center, and it invites visitors to come for a month to experience living and working in this type of community.

Residents and guests live in bungalows and trailers. Daily work tasks include gardening, carpentry, teaching, and weaving. A large conference center seats 1,300 people. There are a day-care center and a kindergarten on the grounds, plus a greenhouse, art studio, and healing center. Independent businesses, such as a drugstore, design studio, and computer company, flourish. Findhorn's successful efforts at gardening on sandy soil in an area with a short growing season and a harsh climate have attracted much interest from around the world.

Policy decisions are made by a core group. Governance also includes input from trustees, a village council, family, and community meetings. Findhorn residents are working toward synergy—individuals knowing their own authority and power and working together to create a whole community. A decision-making process called *attunement* is recognized, in which members meditate on issues and ask for divine guidance, thereby achieving a clear consensus.

Findhorn has been called a "planetary village"—a place where people live connected lives, explore new patterns of cultural and social evolution, and carry their collective vision into other areas of society. They are deeply concerned with the interdependence of all people with the earth and speak of the "global family" and the survival of the planet.

As with many other intentional communities, splinter groups have been formed. A number of people wanting to remain closely connected with Findhorn and its philosophy, and at the same time follow their own initiatives, have chosen an independent membership status. A flourishing group lives in the surrounding area of Forres; twelve people have established a self-supporting village on the Island of Iona; and others, scattered in different countries of the world, have formed their own Findhorn-inspired groups.

One large group of Findhorn "alumni" living on the Pacific coast of North America has developed the Shenoa Retreat Center in Philo, California. *Shenoa* is a native American word meaning "white dove" and refers to the serenity and peace found in nature. This center, two hours north of San Francisco, occupies 160 acres of land. At present, it is not a residential community but a place to gather for inspiration and renewal with other like-minded and like-hearted people. Eighteen cabins and numerous campsites are available, with vegetarian meals served daily in the dining lodge. Weekend or week-long seminars and workshops are presented on such topics as group dynamics, meditation, working with nature, and expressing spiritual values in daily life. People of various racial and economic backgrounds, with different philosophical, religious, and spiritual perspectives are welcomed.

(Interested readers can contact the Shenoa Retreat Center, P.O. Box 43, Philo, California 95466; 707-895-3156.)

Ireland

Our Irish friends Doren and Oisin O'Shiochru decided to build a private annex onto their large home in the small seaside town of Malahide, in County Dublin. They invited Oisin's parents and aunt to live together in the new annex, which is spacious and beautiful, with lots of room for precious old furnishings. Both "homes" were self-sufficient, sharing only a formal backyard garden. Our friends and their four children had their own entrance, as did their older family members.

Each family member was able to follow his or her own life-style, but they shared holiday meals and special celebrations and supported one another in illness, joys, and sorrows. The grandchildren loved having their grandparents close but separate—and our friends felt less anxious about their independent yet aging relatives.

The Middle East

Israel

The Gilo Sheltered Housing Project, Jerusalem

The Gilo project is an experiment in the integration of functionally independent elderly with young families. It is operated under the administration and control of Amidar, a government housing company, which is responsible for maintenance, service, and rent collection.

Fifty-one ground-floor units for older people are distributed among ten four-story residential blocks populated by young middle-class families with children. Home visits and mutual assistance includes the young people's helping the elderly with shopping, garbage disposal, and repair work. The older people reciprocate with baby-sitting and sewing.

Contributing to the success of the project is an on-site housemother, a two-way intercom system, a clinic, and a social club. The staff works at establishing good-neighbor relations among the generations. Local community groups organize intergenerational activities.

For the young, especially those with no living parents or grandparents, this life-style offers a closeness to the older generation. One older woman describes the benefits of the project to her: "I feel part of the young people's lives, and it makes me feel younger to live among them. It is much better than a home for the aging. I want to see young people too, to be part of the community, to have a feeling that life is still exciting."

The Far East

Japan

In Japan, the government provides low-interest loans to people who wish to add a room to their home in order to accommodate an older parent. Housing conditions in general are very poor in Japan, and because of this policy, 74 percent of the elderly live with an adult child.

North America

Canada

Sitka: An Urban Women's Housing Cooperative

The Sitka Housing Cooperative is a landmark—the first women-initiated housing project in British Columbia. It was named "Sitka" for a type of spruce tree that withstands winds better than other evergreens. Sitka was developed by a group of women concerned about the housing crisis and how it affected women whose incomes were so low that they might never be able to afford their own homes. Included in their concerns were women living alone in their old age.

Incorporated as a nonprofit organization in 1982, Sitka hired architect Linda Baker, who felt that women responded to space differently than men. Her architectural plans included larger kitchens connected to living/dining areas, lots of space and light, two-floor apartments, soundproofing, and suite views of courtyards where children could play and people could gather. No two units are the same but are built to reflect the concerns of their occupants. The co-op was specifically designed to fit in with the existing houses on the street—"compatible with the neighbors and gentle within the neighborhood."

The mortgage is insured by the federal government through the Canada Mortgage and Housing Corporation (CMHC). The forty-two women who own and occupy this co-op have become a cohesive, stable group. Intent on living in a caring community, they help each other out with child care, pet-sitting, etc. Everyone takes turns at night to do a security check. Decisions are made by consensus whenever possible.

Residents talk about what it will be like living here in their old age. They have a sense that Sitka is their permanent home, and they expect to grow old here.

The Community Alternatives Society (CAS), Vancouver, British Columbia

In 1979, the Community Alternatives Society's cooperative was opened. More than forty adults and children share this three-story building located on a quiet residential street. The building is divided into nine "pods." Each pod houses groups of three, four, or eight people, and functions as a cooperative house. Each person, child or adult, has his or her own bedroom and shares common spaces with others.

Members of the cooperative range in age from their early thirties to one man in his seventies. Ten members are in their forties and four are in their fifties.

The CAS works as a group toward establishing an egalitarian, nonsexist, intergenerational life-style. They attempt to "live lightly on the land" and close to nature. Celebration and spirituality are recognized as part of life, and political action to create a more humane and equitable society is essential to their philosophy. This community is somewhat like the intentional communities in the United States.

Resident members live either at the co-op or at the ten-acre Fraser Common Farm, which is part of the cooperative, located an hour's drive away. Each resident purchases $2,000 in shares and pays monthly bills by pledge.

The following interview was conducted by a colleague of mine, Martha Tabor, who has a special interest in photographing midlife and older women. She interviewed Kaz Takahashi, a fifty-five-year-old single woman who was part of the original group that formed the Community Alternatives Society.

KAZ TAKAHASHI

When I first joined this group during its early planning stages, I felt that it was really strange. Members were young, and they wanted utopia, and I wanted something much more concrete. It wasn't until two older couples came in that I realized there was a possibility that something could happen. We met every week. It's incredible that we've succeeded.

At that time, I had a house, although I had a student living with me because I didn't like living by myself. While we were waiting for this building to be completed, six of us bought a house together in the interim.

I currently live in an eight-person pod at CAS. Right now I'm taking a break from my work as a public-health nurse and am studying piano and flower arranging. I am the third of five children of Japanese-Canadian parents, and I have lived all of my life in Vancouver (with the exception of eight years in a relocation camp for Japanese-Canadians).

One thing I like about the communal aspect of our living is that I don't have to be the only person making decisions. Whoever lives here has an input, and we try to reach decisions through consensus. It's much easier to deal with problems when there are other people to consult and pass problems through. That's a comfort. The feedback I get from people here, whether it is on an emotional or physical issue, makes me think, "Wow, they really care!"

Here I can work on my constant struggle for sexual equality. I'm learning a lot and am growing personally. I'm learning so

*much more by being in a group than by trying to learn every-
thing through books. I'm now considered an older person, but,
here, aging, like menopause, is no longer a big issue.*

(Interested readers can contact the Community Alternatives Society, 1937 West
Second Avenue, Vancouver, British Columbia, Canada V6J 1J2).

The Pacific

Australia

Bruce Coldham, the architect mentioned in chapter 4, is one of
the American leaders of the cohousing movement. He is a native
of Australia and has had two personal experiences in community
living in Australia before making his home in the United States.
He described them for me in some detail.

A SMALL COLLECTIVE, MELBOURNE

*My first experience in community was a small cohousing com-
munity about a mile from the center of Melbourne. It houses five
families. The children range in age from one to eighteen, and all
the adults are over forty. In the beginning, my family and my
brother's family bought houses next to each other, because we
wanted to share our lives. Now there are five homes sharing a
common road.*

*Spontaneous social-group gatherings take place in our common
yards. Our arrangement really works well in terms of child care,
kid swapping, informal playing by both the children and adults,
and common meals by arrangement. The lower portion of our
big barn serves as a recreation space, especially on rainy or cold
days. Security is tight because we all have a common interest in
surveillance. I remember some bloke trying to break into my
brother's house, when he and his family were away for the weekend. The burglar didn't have a chance.*

*We can prove to people that community living can be fun—
that you get much more than you give.*

The second community experience was when, along with ten families in Australia, we jointly purchased two neighboring houses near Apollo Bay, just two hours from Melbourne. They are used solely for the purpose of developing a shared-vacation community.

We formed a formal cooperative society to acquire the property. Several of us had had some experience in establishing such a collective. One member had been part of a cooperative ski-club society for some years. Each family pays about $3,750 for a share. We decided in the beginning that the community would be oriented towards families rather than singles—that it would be more communal than private. Initially, some building work had to be done to enable four shareholder families (and their friends, by agreement) to live there at the same time, in holiday comfort. An additional input of $350 per family was assessed so that these rearrangements could be made.

We have set up operational rules so that the facilities can be harmoniously used. Space is booked by members by appointment, through one person who has agreed to act as a booking officer. Priorities are set for key holiday periods.

Members contribute a small amount for each day spent here. The income this generates offsets maintenance and service costs. Each member is expected to do their share of maintenance work. Everyone is asked to leave the fireplace set for lighting by the next visiting group and to leave the place tidy.

This really feels like a community, with the only difference being that we don't live there all the time. People spend about 20 percent of the year here—and we have agreed that while we are here, we will spend time together. We have work-party weekends—and we also do things together back in the city. We call ourselves a short-term community. It may not be possible for all of us to live 100 percent of our lives in community, but we can have strong connections for at least part of the time.

Living Close to Family, Australian Style

My daughter Ann, who lives in Mosman, Australia, interviewed an older friend who has arranged her life with both personal privacy and family closeness in mind.

JEAN PATON, BONDI JUNCTION

I am eighty-two years old and for the past three years have lived by myself in a one-bedroom apartment on the eleventh floor of a modern apartment building in Bondi Junction, a small city just outside of Sydney. I immigrated from Scotland to Australia with my husband and two young children thirty-eight years ago.

I was widowed in 1981 and found it increasingly difficult to look after the gardens and large home my husband and I had lived in for more than thirty years. I'm a fiercely independent woman and never even considered living in the same house with either of my daughters. I guard my own precious freedom and never want my children to feel that they are tied down to me. A friend and I started looking into a retirement village near Sydney, but when she decided to move into a flat near her son, my daughter suggested I do the same thing.

I would recommend this living arrangement to everyone.

My daughter Sandra, son-in-law, George, and only grand-daughter (now eighteen years old) live in the same building, just two stories above me. We help each other out whenever we can. Recently, Sandra and her husband were both suffering from disabling injuries, and I pitched in with the cooking and odd jobs. When Sandra and George took off last year for a much-needed holiday, they persuaded me to come along by insisting that they needed me to carry their luggage.

We have our own separate lives but usually manage some time together over the weekends—perhaps a theater evening. During the week, our contact is often limited to telephone conversations. But I feel safe knowing that they are so close. When I lived alone out in the country, I was lonely and often scared and was very concerned about the energy that my busy daughters were spending, driving hours each week to check up on me. I get out and walk briskly for miles every day, usually alone. I find most people my age too elderly and too slow, and it irritates me to walk with them. At least once a week I walk into Sydney, where I go to concerts and to all the museum openings. I volunteer at church once a week and go to the library frequently.

My life is quiet and simple, and that's the way I like it to be. How could anyone be lonely when they can look out at night to the lights of the city and the sea at Botany Bay?

Granny Flats—Privacy with Proximity to Family

The Ministry of Housing in the state of Victoria, Australia, built the first publicly supported "granny flat" in Melbourne in 1975.

Since then, the idea has spread so rapidly that the program has more than 3,000 units in place, with long waiting lists for additional units.

"Granny flats," small, self-contained portable homes designed for easy installation and removal, are placed in the backyard of an adult child or family member. They are prefabricated buildings with a living room, dining room, kitchen, bedroom, and bathroom. Utilities are usually connected to the main house. They are built for one or two older people and are about the size of a two-car garage.

To be eligible for a rental granny flat in Australia, the applicant must receive a pension and have no more than $20,000 in assets; they cannot own a home or have recently sold property. Rental units are moved into the family backyard—and dismantled and moved to a new location to serve another family when they are vacated. Rental agreements are for at least one year's time, and fees are assessed at 20 percent of the applicant's income—or no more than forty-five dollars a week, plus utilities.

People who have more assets are allowed to purchase a unit privately. In that case, the Ministry guarantees that it will buy the unit back at its market value, when it is no longer needed.

A study of the Granny Flat Program in Victoria, conducted by the University of Waterloo, Ontario, Canada (and reported in *The Gerontologist*, Vol. 30, No. 2, 1990), has described a few of the problems that have surfaced during the last decade: The administration of the Granny Flat Program is very time consuming. Program workers experience difficulty in matching an applicant with a home of his or her choice. (In Victoria, there are twenty models of one-bedroom homes and six two-bedroom models. One standardized model has been proposed.) There are often delays in providing the unit and in removing it when it becomes vacant.

However, granny flats are one answer to parental caregiving concerns, offering each family independence and privacy while allowing for frequent interactions and support. Granny flats are being proposed as a helpful tool for single mothers and disabled people as well.

The idea of granny flats is beginning to spread around the world. They are popular in New Zealand, and the Danes call them "kangaroo houses." In England they are called "granny annexes" and are frequently attached to the family home. (This may pose a sale or rental problem when one unit is vacant.) Some annexes are built adjacent to public housing complexes where family members live, allowing an older person to remain in a normal environment and yet have access to services. In rural Sweden, this popular form of housing is called *Stockli*—separate living accommodations for older people added on to the family farmhouse.

In Ontario, Canada, the market study previously mentioned proved that people were ready for the granny flat idea. "Portable Living Units for Seniors" (PLUS) have been successfully built there, as they have been in Alberta. They are often called "garden suites."

This clever housing alternative has not advanced much in the United States because of strict zoning laws. But people are committed to a similar idea called ECHO housing, discussed in chapter 7. Yet, in every country where they exist, granny flats increase opportunities for greater intergenerational understanding.

This is illustrated by Molly Ryan's part-time occupancy of a granny flat. Molly is sixty-seven years old, a widow of eight years, with two adult children who live in Sydney and Melbourne. In her interview with my daughter Ann, she states:

MOLLY RYAN

For the last decade, I've been involved with a few different living arrangements, all of which might be of interest to readers of this book. When my husband was alive, we had a sort of granny flat built on to our home on Danger Island, for our son and daughter and other family members to stay in. After his death, I felt very lonely.

A woman in my debating club, Vicky, who is five years older than me, also lived on her own and was lonely. She suggested that we might give living together a try. She moved into the second flat, so we each had our own complete living quarters. A connecting door joined the two flats.

Living with One Other Person

Rather than living as neighbors, we began to develop a real relationship. Only one television aerial was allowed for the two flats and the TV was in my apartment. We got into the habit of watching it together in the evenings. This worked so well, and we enjoyed each other's company so much, that we decided to have dinner together—each of us cooking every other night. We discovered that we have very different tastes in food, so we began cooking our own meals, having a drink together before dinner, and eating our food as we watched the evening news. Sometimes we just sat and read or talked together.

A year and a half ago, we moved together to another home in the Blue Mountains. We still have our own separate living areas (kitchen, bedroom, and bathroom) in different wings of the house and share a guest bedroom. We have followed the same meal routine, often sitting on our deck together for lunch.

We both love bush-walking, and our relationship has grown to encompass walks together whenever we can. We are both grandparents and share the ups and the downs of our relationships with our children and grandchildren. We love to take holidays together, and do so often. We've traveled to Mexico and Cuba, and right now we are planning a trip to England. Vicky couldn't afford these exotic trips, so I helped pay her expenses, because I don't like traveling alone.

What's been good about our living arrangements is that we like each other, keep each other company, and are interested in each other's lives. There's always someone to talk to about the big occurrences and, more important, the little things that happen on a daily basis. If Vicky had not wanted to move to the Blue Mountains with me, I wouldn't have done it alone.

There are, of course, a few problems. I have been the owner of both of our homes. Vicky has only a small pension and no assets, so she pays a nominal rent. Sometimes I become aware of the fact that the financial and physical burden of home ownership is all on my shoulders.

Our relationship works well because we are of the same generation, have the same standards of cleanliness, and are both relatively tolerant, neither of us being too rigid in our outlook on the world. Both of us are cheerful people who can laugh a lot together, and we have similar political outlooks, although I am definitely the activist. We also share similar interests. Both of us are avid readers, and we love bush-walking. Finally, we both have our own space; the little irritations that arise from living together often start with sharing a kitchen and a bathroom.

My Own "Granny Flat"

Three days of each week, I live in a lovely, large one-room house in my daughter's backyard. Here, I have a comfortable bed, a dining and kitchen area, and a small bathroom.

I come down to Sydney every Thursday and stay until Saturday morning. This gives me time to visit with friends and with my family. I pick up my two grandsons from after-school care, so that they can have one day a week to come home and play. I also cook our dinners, and we all eat together.

We built this house when I was living on isolated Danger Island. There were no cars allowed on the island, and few services were available. My family was worried about what would happen when I could no longer cope with this type of daily living. Now, with Vicky and me living together in the Blue Mountains, the whole idea of the house is less relevant.

Chapter Nine

Living Alone or as a Couple: Life-styles with a Twist

Midlife and older people are experimenting with a wide variety of life-styles. Many older people live alone in a traditional fashion. Others design unique living situations to meet their needs for housing with adventure.

Life at Sea

One innovative woman spends ten months a year on freighters, sailing around the world and returning to visit relatives and friends during the summer. She uses her federal pension and a small social-security check to finance her ocean-going adventures. It costs her about $6,000 for ten months at sea, compared to $2,000 for her two-month home stays. At age seventy she boarded a Polish freighter for a cruise to the Far East, saying, "For me, there is no better way to find absolute freedom from responsibility or worry than getting on a freighter and sailing wherever the ship will take me. And I make new friends on every trip, meeting people I ordinarily would never have a chance to meet."

Two women, age sixty-two and sixty-five, have been sailing on freighters for several years, and they love it. A friend of ours sent us their Christmas-greeting letter, which is mailed to family and friends, from wherever they are in the world.

> This was a great year. We shipped out of Houston in May. The two-month trip down the east coast of South America was delightful. Back to the United States to spend two months in Nova Scotia and with family. In November we will fly to Brussels, then on to Hamburg. Early in December we will board a German freighter for a four-month trip around the world. It's a nine-passenger cargo ship, which stops in five ports in England and France. Then we'll be going across the Atlantic, through the Panama Canal, and on south to Tahiti; Fiji; Samoa; Papua, New Guinea; Guadalcanal; and any other ports where freight must be picked up. Home via Singapore, across the Indian Ocean, through the Suez Canal, with a stop in Spain before returning to Rotterdam. Then we plan to lease a car for three or four months and do some touring in Portugal, Spain, England, Wales, and Scotland. In midsummer we are booked for a mail-boat trip up the coast of Norway. We are planning mail-calls four or five times in our ten-month odyssey and would love to hear from you. We're having a great time roaming around.

Life Overseas

Volunteer Services

Some midlife and older people join the Peace Corps and head for foreign countries to offer volunteer services. Others join VISTA and help needy people in the United States.

A friend of mine in her late seventies has recently joined the Peace Corps in Poland, to teach English to Polish business-people. A couple I know, now in their late fifties, plan to retire soon, and bring their talents and skills (he is a physician and she is a nurse/social worker/bereavement counselor) to one of the Peace Corps countries.

I talked by phone to Charles (sixty-six) and Margaret Harmon (sixty-five) from Cushing, Minnesota. Beginning in 1985, they spent two years in the Peace Corps, in Jamacia, and are heading out for their second assignment next month—this time to the Carribean island of Saint Lucia.

Margaret and Charles have been married forty-four years and have five adult children and seven grandchildren. They have lived for twenty years in a big log house on one of Minnesota's many lakes; before then they farmed, and codirected a Bible camp.

It has been their long-time dream to help people in the Third World. In Jamaica, Charles used his degree in animal husbandry, working with the men of a small dairy farm co-op. Margaret worked with people of all ages in the 4H and initiated a rural town's first library. They lived in an all-cement home in a government housing project with the people they worked with—and made many good friends who call or write to them often. They say:

> We're returning to the Peace Corps, because we have learned what we can do—and that there are lots of places in the world where we are needed. We feel pride in having accomplished something worthwhile. As you grow older in this country, you are not needed, and all too often you are forced to fill your time with travel, restaurants, and shopping. In the Peace Corps, when we were done with our work each day, we had had a new experience, and we had helped someone. We're really excited about our next new experience.

Retiring Overseas

An adventuresome couple from suburban New York wrote the following to the editor of a major newspaper:

> My husband (a vigorous, young sixty-eight) and myself (ditto, fifty-eight) have just sold our co-op in preparation for retirement in the south of France. Our five children live all around the country. We are free to go; we don't want to be in any of their backyards. They are very welcome to spend Christmas and part of the summer with us. Now it's our turn. We love all the children fiercely—especially with the Atlantic Ocean between us.

Living in Two Different Worlds

I interviewed one of my dear old friends, Elisabeth MacKenzie (Mac), whose life-style I find intriguing. The interview took place on her ninetieth birthday, in the small town of Middlefield, Massachusetts.

ELISABETH MACKENZIE

For thirty years I worked and lived with a woman friend who died when I was seventy-four. Our lives were rich—we spent six months in a small cabin in the woods of rural Massachusetts and six months during the winters in our home next to the water in Fort Lauderdale, Florida. I've managed to continue that life-style alone, for more than sixteen years. I bought a Winnebago bus, which keeps me very busy going on trips to every one of the United States.

The two places I live in are quite different. In each I have a trained guard dog living with me that offers tremendous protection and good company. My house in Florida backs onto a beautiful canal and is next door to my brother. I belong to three Winnebago clubs, the United States Power Squadron Auxiliary, the Appalachian Mountain Association, and the American Legion. I always go to the Orange Bowl festivities and attend the theater often.

My home in the middle of the woods in Massachusetts is small and compact, near a beautiful waterfall. When I arrive each May, my calendar begins to fill up rapidly, with friends inviting me to dinner, church suppers, senior-citizen luncheons, and the annual country fair. I belong to the Middlefield Grange and the Concerned Citizens and go to church every Sunday. Lots of my family and friends visit me here—and since I really don't know how to cook, we're always going out to dinner. Since I've been alone, a friend of mine in Middlefield calls me up at eight o'clock every morning to see if I'm okay. By the time October rolls around, my friends from Florida are calling me to see when I am coming home.

On the whole, my life has been perfectly happy. I've met so many interesting people and hope to continue meeting more. I know that I'm lucky to have enough money to live in two totally different environments. And I still feel that there's a great deal more that I want to get out of life. I'm not about to roll over and die.

Another friend, Joan Strohschnitter, who was recently widowed also spends her year in two totally different parts of the country.

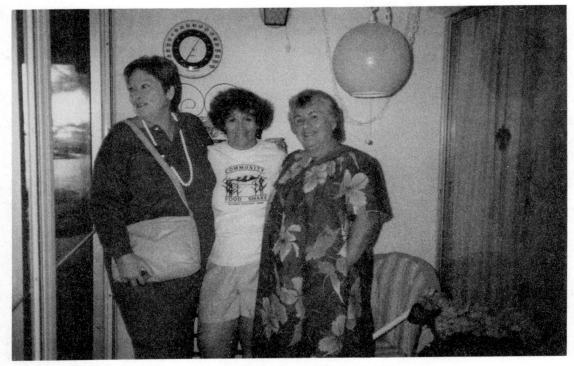

Joan Strohschnitter at home in Deerfield Beach, Florida, with Eileen Wengler and Barbara Paldino.

JOAN STROHSCHNITTER

A year and a half after Charlie's death, I knew I needed a change. Just at that point, some friends I had played tennis with several years before called from Florida. Thirteen of these women had bought units in the same condominium in Deerfield Beach. They assured me that a unit had just been put on the market and was meant for me, so I made reservations to fly down to see it. It took only two days to make my decision, and the contract was signed. All I had to do was sell my home and move out thirty-six years' accumulation of junk. I hired a garage-sale specialist (my sister, June) who sold thirteen tons of gorgeous, valuable, and irreplaceable items. Another forty-nine truckloads of memorable acquisitions were carted out and shoved into my little cabin in Wading River. Now it is impossible to open the cabin door without a great deal of heaving and hauling.

My new unit is just twenty feet from the waterway. Every

morning I walk over to the ocean and watch the sun rise. I go swimming with friends most days, joined a shuffleboard group, attend the harness races, and signed for a luncheon cruise. I love seeing my first live alligator, blue herons, and egrets.

I travel north with the other "snow birds" in May—to live again near the beach in a familiar little cabin I have summered in for more than thirty years. Hopefully, my nephew Chris will spend most of the summer with me. In Florida there are new friends and new sights—in Wading River, my solid old friends and family await me. It's a good life.

Bringing "The World" to Your Home

Strawberry Farm Bed and Breakfast

Our family has a small A-frame house in the woods of Massachusetts, where we spend summers and as many weekends as possible. Among our friends in this tiny town of Middlefield are Judy and Vic Artioli. Judy returned to the University of Massachusetts when the youngest of her six children was still little. Four years later, she won high honors and awards for her paintings and folk-art sculptures. Her art is being shown at many popular galleries in the Northeast. In a few years, we will be saying, "We knew her when!"

Despite having a large and active family, living and painting in a tiny community of 350 people could have been very lonely for Judy. However, Judy decided to open up three rooms of their home as a bed and breakfast. This is her story:

JUDY ARTIOLI

Running a bed and breakfast for the past few years has taken away some of the isolation we felt in living in a small town in New England.

We advertise in brochures for tourists who want to visit the Northeast and are members of the Hampshire Bed and Breakfast Association. That group has a yearly dinner meeting, and we act as a wonderful network for one another. When one of us is "full," we recommend one of the others in the association. Our ad reads:

Strawberry Farm—An Artist's Residence—Lush, pastoral views surround us in this restored 1780 farmhouse. Original paintings and art are displayed. Homemade breads and other goodies, including gourmet fresh-ground coffee, are served.

Would you believe that some people tell us it was the coffee and homemade breads that caught their eye? Most people stay two days and frequently come back the following year; one hunter has been coming to spend a week every December for the past five years. Our guests seem to like the personal environment and the art surrounding them. We've had three sets of honeymooners, therapists, bankers, physicians, writers, artists—people from many walks of life.

After a hard day's work, my husband finds it very relaxing to have people to chat with in the evening. At first, our six teenagers were shy and reluctant to talk to strangers, but now they love it too—and they have learned so much about the world. Guests talk to me while I'm making breakfast, and we have long conversations about my paintings and sculptures (which they often purchase).

We have people coming from all over—India and Turkey, Oregon and California; the world seems to be coming to our doorstep, enriching all of us who live here.

(Interested readers can contact Judy and Vic Artioli, Strawberry Farm, Middlefield, Massachusetts 02142.)

I admire the adventuresome, vital people described in this chapter, for not "settling" for life—not repeatedly choosing the old familiar routine. They have struck out for new territory, taken risks and more chances. They have used the gifts of health and extra years to discover new people, new talents, and new interests—and they all seem to be happier as a result.

Epilogue:

The Shape of Things to Come

The reality is clear. Most of us will want to—or need to—make some type of housing adjustment in our later years. That's what this book is all about. It has identified some of the community-type housing options—from the traditional retirement village to the intentional community; from age-segregated to intergenerational shared housing; from an all-female home to homes with mixed genders and ages; from all single people to those who choose to live with other couples and families; from those who are relatively poor to those who are wealthy. Today, people in their forties, fifties, sixties, and seventies are more open than ever before to new lifestyles, new households, and new housing.

Despite—or even because of—serious government neglect in the eighties (including an 85 percent cut in low-income housing), housing for the rapidly growing number of midlife and older people is one of the most pressing concerns facing the country in the next decade.

The Reality

People are really concerned about future housing! In the years since I wrote the chapter on housing in *Growing Older, Getting Better*, I have had mail from all over the country.

> Increasingly, I have been developing an awareness of the need for new living arrangements/life-styles. Like many others my age, I have been experiencing social and economic insecurity. I feel very lucky to be a woman in the second stage of my life—and I have tremendous vitality and joie de vivre. The idea of community has been taking root in my heart for several years, but how do I start?
> Virginia Altmann, Medford, Massachusetts

> I am a widow in my sixties, working and living alone. I have excellent references and am in good health. As an independent person, I would like to be living where I could be paying a more reasonable rent for my income—and where I could be with people who were keeping an eye out for one another.
> Betty Diture, Arlington, Virginia

> What we desperately need for our own sanity and contentment are living arrangements whereby we have our own quarters but also the contact of other people. We need arrangements that are simple and inexpensive. Most of us are just getting by—and there are more of us every year. Please help.
> Marguerite Arnold, Dedham, Massachusetts

> Please hurry up with your book on housing options! My husband has a severe heart condition, which forces me to think ahead. I'm forty-five and know that I don't want to live alone. I want privacy along with accessibility to other interesting, activist people—and a social life. One thing I know is that I don't want to live with any of my kids!
> Anonymous, New York City, New York

> What we need to do is educate planners, housing advocates, politicians, and governments about the im-

portance of understanding the "social" meaning of housing. Shelter is more than four walls and a roof over one's head. It is the nest, the home-port of family wellness; it is from this safe place that we can face the world.

Edwina Fong, Honolulu, Hawaii

Unfortunately, few of us have done much planning for our future housing needs. The 1990 AARP survey, which I refer to in the introduction, showed that 35 percent of those fifty-five and older had done no planning *at all*, and another 18 percent had done *little* planning. Those who had begun planning were usually married, in the fifty-five to sixty-four age bracket, and home owners with annual incomes of $36,000 or more.

As I lecture around the country, it becomes clear that people are still very fearful that their future housing choices are limited. They've only heard of three options: staying on in their own underutilized home, moving to a retirement village, or being placed in a nursing home. But more and more people want to live the second half of their lives in or near urban areas—to take advantage of good transportation systems in a full cultural environment. And most people want to live close enough to their adult children or other relatives to visit on a weekly or bi-weekly basis.

Women, who are much more likely to be living longer, living alone, and unable to afford market-rate housing, especially are concerned about future housing. Living in family homes that are much too large for them, many women are "house rich" and money poor. They stay put in their "mismatched" homes, because they are unaware of the alternatives. Many of them would welcome aid to help locate a home more suitable to their present circumstances and needs.

This is the first book written about and for the eighty-five percent of aging people who are in good health, and who want to live to their fullest potential. Most of the current literature about housing and the elderly is written about the 15 percent of older people who are frail or near-frail.

The Good News

The interviews for this book have had me crisscrossing the country, meeting with hundreds of zestful midlife and older people. I've discovered that people in their sixties and seventies are not settling for less than ideal housing, nor permanent ("until I die") arrangements. They see their present life-styles as "good for now," but they're challenged to continue to explore and move on to something better if and when it comes along.

I've also found that there is a growing variety of housing options to meet the needs of the rapidly growing midlife and older population, especially for those who are well and independent. And, according to the AARP, one option that is particularly growing in popularity is shared housing. More than 76 percent of those surveyed by the AARP said they preferred living in a neighborhood with people of all ages rather than in an age-segregated neighborhood. Half of the respondents (both single and married) would consider some form of shared housing.

Since a growing number of us "young-olds" are financially able to choose from one of the traditional or alternative housing options (because we have accumulated twenty-or thirty-year equity in our family home), let's begin to plan ahead! Let's not put off housing action until some sort of health or financial crisis arrives, and let's not risk letting someone else make these important decisions for us as we age!

The Government's Role in the Decades Ahead

A crucial need in housing for older Americans is the resumption of strong support on the federal level, to enable those who wish to remain in their own homes to obtain adequate social and supportive services, and to develop a wide range of housing alternatives for people of all income levels.

The National Institute of Senior Housing (NISH) foresees housing preferences and needs of the baby-boom generation as quite different from those of their parents and grandparents. The new elderly are likely to be more actively involved in politics and to be more assertive with respect to how and where they want to live.

A pilot program begun by the *Federal National Mortgage Association* will expand housing options for those sixty-two or over. Four types of loans will be available to finance accessory apartments (self-contained units built as part of a single-family residence), ECHO cottages, one-to-one homesharing, and sale-leaseback (in which an older person sells their home to a relative or investor who then leases it back, allowing the seller to gain from the sale proceeds while remaining in the same house).

Zoning Deregulation. The emergence of zoning laws in 1920 restricted multifamily housing in newly developing suburbs; now, the suburbs have become a sea of single-family homes. A new trend (called *housing deregulation* or *up-zoning*) has begun to reverse the strict zoning laws, allowing for the construction of small, low-income, owner-occupied multifamily housing. Albany, New York, has begun building new two-family row homes, and Boston is allowing the first new construction of three-family homes since 1920.

We're On Our Way

My goal is to see the achievement of a diverse array of imaginatively financed and redesigned homes for midlife and older people. Clearly, housing must offer security, economy, and community.

In writing this book, I have begun to uncover a host of exciting housing possibilities. I am advocating choices in living arrangements and choices in housing—in short, choices for living better. As one woman I know puts it: "To be thinking about a new way to live at age fifty is not a burden, it's an adventure."

We are living longer than people have ever lived before, and with that comes the challenge to live better. Gail Godwin, in her novel *The Finishing School,* says:

> Really, aging is not the enemy—nor is death. We ought to fear the kind of death that happens in life. Some people stop growing, learning, or changing . . . they *congeal!* And even though they may be perfectly nice people, you can expect no more surprises from them. Another kind of person is fluid, keeps moving forward, making new trysts with life. They are alive, and fun to be with.

Together, let's continue the search for innovative and creative housing options for midlife and older Americans. This book is only a beginning. In explaining, describing, and questioning the successes of several present housing options, we are beginning to make statements, implicit or explicit, about the quality of life wanted by all people in their middle years and beyond; about the need for change; the content of our recent legislation; the very nature of a new generation of healthy and vigorous older people. Discussions have been revitalized, and policies and potential options are being viewed from a new and different perspective.

We will all benefit from the sharing of ideas in this area. I am beginning to notice an enthusiastic exploration of and a new openness in communication about a wide scope of community-housing options that are available today. People are being asked to share their ideas and experiences; articles directly invite comment; networks are being created; newsletters are being circulated to extend support. The vulnerability of not knowing what the future will bring for older Americans is becoming a shared experience.

Older people are growing in number and in power, and most of us are staying healthy right to the end. We are searching for a zestful old age—and know that *who* we live with and *where* we live, will contribute to the quality of our lives.

The women and men I have met and interviewed as I traveled around this country and abroad have definitely not congealed. They have enriched my life by being so fully alive—and I suspect that each of them is not only living longer, but living better.

Bibliography
and Resources

Small-Group Living

Books

Branwein, Nancy; MacNeice, Jill; and Spiers, Peter. *The Group House Handbook.* Washington, DC: Acropolis Books, 1982.

Hanaway, Lorraine, ed. *The 3-in-1 House.* Home Care Research (30 East Patrick Street, Frederick, MD 21701), 1981.

Horne, Jo, with Leo Baldwin. *Home-Sharing and Other Life-style Options.* Washington, DC: AARP, 1988.

Jaffe, Dale. *Shared Housing for the Elderly.* Westport, CT: Greenwood Press, 1989.

Pastalan, Leon, and Cowart, Marie. *Life-styles and Housing of Older Adults: The Florida Experience.* New York: Haworth Press, 1989.

Peace, Sheila, and Nusberg, Charlotte. *Shared Living: A Viable Alternative for the Elderly.* Washington, DC: International Federation on Aging, 1984.

Raimy, Eric. *Shared Houses, Shared Lives: The New Extended Families and How They Work.* Los Angeles: J. P. Tarcher, Inc., 1979.

Streib, Gordon; Folts, Edward; and Hilker, Mary Anne. *Old Homes—New Families: Shared Living for the Elderly.* New York: Columbia University Press, 1984.

Resources

Booklets, films, and slides available from the Community Services Department, Action for Boston Community Development (ABCD) Inc., 178 Tremont Street, Boston, MA 02111:

Planning and Developing a Shared Living Project: A Guide for Community Groups.
Shared Living: A Community Planning Guide.
Shared Living: An Individual Planning Guide.

Film: *Open House: Shared Living for Older People.*
Slide show/discussion guide: *Families of Choice.*

Ecumenical Association for Housing, 1510 5th Avenue, San Rafael, CA 94915.

National Shared Housing Resource Center, 6344 Greene Street, Philadelphia, PA 19144:

Planning Manual for Group Residencies.
Planning Manual for Match-up Programs.

Women's Search for Housing

Books

Birch, Eugenie. *The Unsheltered Woman: Women and Housing in the 80s.* New Brunswick, NJ: Center for Urban Policy Research, Rutgers University, 1985.

Cheney, Joyce, ed. *Lesbian Land.* Minneapolis, MN: Word Weavers, 1985.

Doress, Paula; Siegal, Diana; and The Midlife and Older Women Book Project. *Ourselves Growing Older: Women Aging with Knowledge and Power.* New York: Simon and Schuster, 1987.

Porcino, Jane. *Growing Older, Getting Better: A Handbook for Women in the Second Half of Life.* Reading, MA: Addison-Wesley, 1983.

Resources

Lesbian Connection. Bi-monthly newsletter about lesbian communities (Helen Diner Memorial Women's Center, P.O. Box 811, East Lansing, MI 48826).

Women's Design Service (WDS). Publishes *Women and the Built Environment,* a quarterly magazine focusing on innovations in planning for women. 62 Beechwood Road, London EB 3DY.

Women and Environments. A magazine published by the Centre for Urban and Community Studies, 455 Spadina Avenue, Toronto, Ontario M5S 2G8.

Women's Housing Coalition. N.Y.C. Commission on the Status of Women, (212-796-7950).

Cohousing

Books

McCamant, Kathryn, and Durrett, Charles. *Cohousing: A Contemporary Approach to Housing Ourselves.* Berkeley, CA: Habitat Press, 1988.

McCamant, Kathryn, and Durrett, Charles. "Cohousing in Denmark," in Franck, Karen, and Ahrentzen, Sherry, *New Households, New Housing*. New York: Van Nostrand Reinhold, 1989.

Resources

The CoHousing Company, 48 Shattuck Square, Suite 15, Berkeley, CA 94704 (415-549-9980). National referral network, to connect interested people throughout the country. They offer a weekend workshop entitled "Getting Started," which includes a slide presentation called *Introducing the CoHousing Concept.*

McCamant and Durett's book is available ($21.45), as are regional contact lists ($10) for areas in the country in which people have expressed an interest in living in a cohousing community.

The CoHousing Newsletter Quarterly. Innovative Housing, 325 Doherty Drive, Larkspur, CA 94939. $20/individuals, $30/organizations for two-year subscription.
Northeast Cohousing Quarterly: A Forum for the Development of Cohousing Communities in the Northeast and Mid-Atlantic States. 155 Pine Street, Amherst, MA 01002. $10/individuals, $25/organizations for one-year subscription.
Cohousing Clearing House of Greater Boston. Promotes the idea of cohousing at regular meetings, from which core groups form. Call Jeff Frie, 617-629-2432.

Large Intentional Communities

Books

Campbell, Susan. *Earth Community*. San Francisco: Evolutionary Press, 1983.
Fromm, Dorit. *Collaborative Communities: A New Concept of Housing with Shared Services*. San Rafael, CA: Ecumenical Association for Housing, 1988.
McLaughlin, Corinne, and Davidson, Gordon. *Builders of the Dawn: Community Lifestyles in a Changing World*. Shutesbury, MA: Sirius Publishing, 1986.
Popenoe, Cris, and Popenoe, Oliver. *Seeds of Tomorrow*. San Francisco: Harper and Row, 1984.

Resources

Communities Magazine. 127 Sun Street, Stelle, IL 60919.

Traditional Housing Options

Books

Carlin, Vivian, and Mansberg, Ruth. *Where Can Mom Live? A Family Guide to Living Arrangements for Elderly Parents.* Indianapolis: Lexington Books, 1987.

————. *If I Live to Be 100: Congregate Housing for Later Life.* West Nyack, NY: Parker, 1984.

Gold, Margaret. *Guide to Housing Alternatives for Older Citizens.* Mount Vernon, NY: Consumers Union, 1985.

Lawton, Powell, and Hoover, Sally, eds. *Community Housing Choices for Older Americans.* New York: Springer-Verlag, 1981.

Resources

Booklets, films, and slides available from the American Association of Retired Persons (AARP), 1909 K Street, N.W., Washington, DC 20049:

The Continuing-Care Retirement Community: A Guidebook for Consumers.

ECHO Housing: A Review of Zoning Issues and Other Considerations.

Housing Options for Older Americans.

A Model Ordinance for ECHO Housing.

1988 National Continuing Care Directory (second edition).

Planning Your Retirement Housing.

Understanding Senior Housing for the 1990s: An American Association of Retired Persons Survey of Consumer Preferences, Concerns, and Needs.

Your Home, Your Choice: A Workbook for Older People and Their Families.

Slide/tape presentation: *ECHO Housing.*

Consumer Housing Information Service for Seniors (CHISS). The AARP trains senior housing information aides to provide information to older consumers about housing options and services available in their communities.

A Consumer Guide to Life-Care Communities. Published by the National Consumers League, Washington, DC.

Continuing-Care Retirement Communities: An Industry in Action.

Published by the American Association of Homes for the Aging, 1129 20th Street N. W., Washington, DC 20036.
Housing the Elderly Report. A monthly newsletter published by CD Publications, 8555 16th Street, Silver Spring, MD.

General Housing and Community Living

Books

Committee on an Aging Society, Institute of Medicine. *The Social and Built Environment in an Older Society.* Washington, DC: National Academy of Sciences Press, 1988.

Dychtwald, Ken, with Flower, Joe. *Age Wave: The Challenges and Opportunities of an Aging America.* Los Angeles: J. P. Tarcher, 1989.

Felder, David. *The Best Investment: Land in a Loving Community.* Tallahassee, FL: Wellington Press, 1982.

Hancock, J. A., ed. *Housing the Elderly.* New Brunswick, NJ: Center for Urban Policy Research, Rutgers University, 1987.

Hayden, Dolores. *Redesigning the American Dream: The Future of Housing, Work and Family Life.* New York: Norton, 1984.

Institute for Community Economics. *The Community Trust Handbook.* Emmaus, PA: Rodale Press, 1982.

Katsura, Harold; Struyk, Raymond; and Newman, Sandra. *Housing for the Elderly in 2010: Projections and Policy Options.* Washington, DC: Urban Institute Press, 1990.

Marcus, Clare Cooper, and Sarkissian, Wendy. *Housing As If People Mattered: Site Design Guidelines for Medium-Density Family Housing.* Berkeley: University of California Press, 1987.

Martin, Thomas, et al. *Adaptive Use: Development, Economics, Process and Profiles.* Washington, DC: Urban Land Institute, 1978.

Peck, M. Scott. *A Different Drummer: Community Making and Peace.* New York: Simon and Schuster, 1987.

Raschko, Betty Ann. *Housing Interiors for the Disabled and Elderly.* New York: Van Nostrand Reinhold, 1982.

Regnier, Victor, and Pynoos, Jon, eds. *Housing the Aged: Design Directives and Policy Considerations.* New York: Elsevier Science, 1987.

Urban Land Institute. *Housing for a Maturing Population.* Washington, DC: American Institute of Architects, 1983.

Yankelovich, Daniel. *New Rules: Searching for Self-Fulfillment in a World Turned Upside Down.* New York: Random House, 1981.

Resources

Journal of Housing for the Elderly. Haworth Press, 28 East 22nd Street, New York, NY 10010.

National Policy Center on Housing and Living Arrangements for Older Americans, University of Michigan, Ann Arbor, MI 48109.

Index